Antidiabet   ...as Pinnata

Shabana Khatoon

Antidiabetic activity on Spondias Pinnata

LAP LAMBERT Academic Publishing

Imprint

Any brand names and product names mentioned in this book are subject to trademark, brand or patent protection and are trademarks or registered trademarks of their respective holders. The use of brand names, product names, common names, trade names, product descriptions etc. even without a particular marking in this work is in no way to be construed to mean that such names may be regarded as unrestricted in respect of trademark and brand protection legislation and could thus be used by anyone.

Cover image: www.ingimage.com

Publisher:
LAP LAMBERT Academic Publishing
is a trademark of
International Book Market Service Ltd., member of OmniScriptum Publishing Group
17 Meldrum Street, Beau Bassin 71504, Mauritius

Printed at: see last page
ISBN: 978-613-9-95451-3

Zugl. / Approved by: Integral university

Antidiabetic activity of *Spondias Pinnata*

against Streptozocin induced diabetes in rats

By: SHABANA KHATOON
(M.Pharm Pharmacology)
Integral university
Lucknow

Acknowledgement

All praises and thanks are for the "One Universal Being and the creator of this universe" who enlightened my life with the light of knowledge and for providing enough patience, self-inspiration and strength that enable me to complete this thesis successfully.

Some wonderful people in this world helped me to pursue my study and I would like to thank all of them. It is my privilege to express my deep sense of gratitude to **Prof S.W. Akthar**, Vice Chancellor, Integral University, and **Dr. T. Usmani**, acting Pro Vice Chancellor, Integral University, as well as **Prof. S.M. Iqbal**, Chief Academic Consultant, Integral University, for providing infrastructure and facilities required for this research work in the Department of Pharmacology, Faculty of Pharmacy, Integral University, Lucknow.

It is my pleasure to express my deep sense of gratitude and thankfulness to my honourable Supervisor **Prof. (Dr) H.H.Siddhiqui,** Advisor to Vice Chancellor, Faculty of Pharmacy, Integral University, Lucknow, for his able cooperative guidance, constant support, patience and encouragement at each and every stage throughout my thesis work. His wide knowledge and his logical way of thinking have been of great value for me. He provided me the excellent advice that has been helpful during the preparation of this thesis despite his busy academic schedules.

I would like to express my deep and humble regards to my Co-Supervisor, **(Dr.) Md. Talib Hussain,** Department of Pharmacology, for invigorates guidance, felicitous advice, punctilious and valuable hints with energizing, criticism, thought during the course of my research work. Indeed without his guidance and optimistic approach this project wouldn't have been a successful one.

I would like to acknowledge whole heartily to my Co-Supervisor **Dr. Chandana Venkateswara Rao,** Senior Scientist, Department of Pharmacology, National Botanical Research Institute (NBRI-CSIR), Lucknow, for helping me throughout the study, in terms of constant support and guidance to define, expand, and explore new knowledge as part of this thesis.

I am deeply indebted to our HOD, **Dr. Jubair Akhtar**, Faculty of Pharmacy, Integral University, for his support and help to carry out this research work.

I am greatly indebted to **Dr. M. Vijay Kumar**, Scientist-C, Pharmacognosy and Ethnopharmacology Division, NBRI encouraged me from time to time and offered guidance in writing the thesis.

I wish to owe special thanks to my friends **Ayyub, Mukim, Muazzam, Ishtiyaq and Hina ,Monika** for their support and continued encouragement to do quality work.

I would also like to thank **Mr. Rashid Siddiqui,** and **Mrs. Barnali Bose**, for their immense help to my work in various ways.

I am cordially grateful to my beloved **parents Mr.Jameel Ahmad,Mrs.Shoaiba Khatoon** and my siblings **Shabeeha Khatoon, Rahmat ali, Murshida Khatoon,** who always covered me under the shade of their love and blessings for their valuable moral support directly or indirectly, the spirit and cooperation for the timely completion of my research work.I cannot forget the support lended to me by **Mr.Rafiuddin,**my husband and two little angles **Mohd. Tanzeel,Samaira Fatima** along with my in laws.

My special thanks to my friend **Shazia Usmani** and **Mohd. Arif.**

My work is the result of prayers and blessings of my mother and hard work of my father enabling me to reach this point of my career. Also I want to thank all of those, whom I may not be able to name individually, for helping me in anyway.

SHABANA KHATOON

LIST OF ABBREVIATIONS

ALP	:	Alkaline phosphatase .
ALT	:	Alanine transminases AST
	:	Aspartate transaminase
BUN	:	Blood nitrogen urea CAT
	:	Catalase
CCl_4	:	Carbon tetrachloride. CMC
	:	Carboxymethylcellulose
G6Pase	:	Glucose 6:phosphatase. GPx
	:	Glutathione peroxidase GSH
	:	Reduced gluthathione GST
	:	Glutathione S: transferase Hb
	:	Haemoglobin
i.p.	:	Intraperitoneal
	:Per oral	
RBC	:	Red blood cells
R_f	:	Retention factor
RNA	:	Ribonucleic acid
SGOT	:	Serum glutamic oxaloacetic transaminase SGPT
	:	Serum glutamic pyruvate transaminase.
SOD	:	Super oxide Dismutase TP
	:	Total Protein
SPE	:	Spondias pinnata extract
STZ	:	Streptozocin
GLB	:	Glibenclamide

(1.1.1) INTRODUCTION:

The world prevalence of diabetes in 2010 among adults aged 20-79 years is estimated to 6.4%, affecting 285 million adults. Between 2010 and 2030, there is an expected 70% increase in numbers of adults with diabetes in developing countries and a 20% increase in developed countries. Each year more than 231,000 people in the United states and more than 3,96 million people worldwide die from diabetes and its complications. This number is expected to increase by more than 50 percent over next decade. (Arunachalam et al., 2013). According to W.H.O. report, the present number of diabetics worldwide is 150 million and is likely to increase to 300 million or more by the year 2025. The worldwide prevalence of diabetes mellitus (DM) has risen dramatically over the past two decade, based on current trends, more than 360 million individuals will have diabetes by year 2030 (Berbecaru-Iovan et al., 2009).

Table -1 *Top 10 countries for numbers of people aged 20-79 years with diabetes in2010 and 2030*

	2010		2030	
	Country	No. of adults with diabetes (millions)	Country	No. of adults with diabetes (millions)
1	India	50.8	India	87.0
2	China	43.2	China	62.6
3	USA	26.8	USA	36.0
4	Russian Federation	9.6	Pakistan	13.8
5	Brazil	7.6	Brazil	12.7
6	Germany	7.5	Indonesia	12.0
7	Pakistan	7.1	Mexico	11.9
8	Japan	7.1	Bangladesh	10.4
9	Indonesia	7.0	Russian Federation	10.3
10	Mexico	6.8	Egypt	8.6

(1.1.2) Defination

Diabetes mellitus is a metabolic disease that occurs either when the pancreas does not produce enough insulin or when the body cannot effectively use the insulin it produces. Insulin is a hormone that regulates blood sugar. Defective insulin secretion is the major cause for chronic hyperglycemia resulting in impaired function or serious damage to many of the body systems like eyes, kidneys, nerves, heart and blood vessels.

(1.1.3) Recent Diabetic Medicine:

Recent Diabetes Medicine Approvals New medicines approved by the FDA in the last year represent exciting steps forward in efforts to better treat diabetes. These include: Nesina (alogliptin) is a new DPP-4 inhibitor designed to slow the inactivation of incretin hormones GLP-1 and GIP, resulting in more active incretins enabling the pancreas to secrete insulin and better managing blood glucose levels. Invokana (canagliflozin) is the first sodium-glucose cotransporter 2 (SGLT2) inhibitor approved for patients with type 2 diabetes. SGLT2 inhibitors work in conjunction with the kidneys and the natural urination process to remove excess blood glucose from the body. Duetact (pioglitazone/glimepiride) combines two previously approved type 2 diabetes medicines with complementary actions in a single tablet. One medicine targets insulin resistance while the other increases the amount of insulin produced by the pancreas. 2 Farxiga (dapagliflozin) is a new SGLT2 inhibitor approved to improve glycemic control in adults with type 2 diabetes. Next-Generation Oral Treatment a medicine in development for the treatment of type 2 diabetes is part of the DPP-4 inhibitor class, but chemically distinct from other approved medicines in this class. DPP-4 inhibitors work by stimulating the production of insulin and producing less glucose. In clinical trials, the medicine was able to inhibit more than 80 percent of its target enzyme for seven days, making it potentially a once-weekly treatment versus daily. Once-Weekly Treatment—A medicine in development is in the same class of drugs as some other approved medicines for type 2 diabetes, but with a longer therapeutic life.

(1.1.3.1) Types of diabetes:

There are four main types of diabetes mellitus.(Patel et al., 2012).

(a) Type   1.   diabetes   (or)   insulin   dependent   diabetes   mellitus

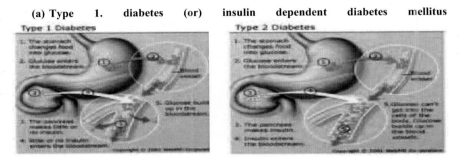

Fig.1a   Fig.1b.

Earlier known as insulin dependent diabetes mellitus (IDDM) or juvenile-onset diabetes mellitus. People with this type of diabetes make little or no insulin in their body, and need regular insulin injections for survival and management of diabetes. It usually starts in childhood, but can occur at any age. This may be immune mediated or idiopathic.

+ **Immune mediated DM**: This result from a cellular mediated autoimmune destruction of the   cells of pancreas, leading to absolute insulin deficiency.

The intrinsic factors that cause immune mediated DM is genetic susceptibility linked to two genes on chromosome 6. These genes control the productions of Human Leukocyte Antigens s(HLAs) DR3,DR4 and people with either (or) both of these antigens have a greater chance of developing DM than a person lacking them.

The extrinsic factors that may lead to immune mediated DM are viruses such as Mumps or Coxsackie B4 (i.e., β-cell cytotoxic) virus leads to release of destructive cytotoxins and antibodies released by sensitized lymphocytes and also by auto digestion in the course of an inflammatory disorder involving the exocrine pancreas.

Markers of immune destruction of β-cells are Islet cell Antibodies (ICAs),Insulin Auto Antibodies (IAAs),Auto Antibodies to Glutamic acid decarboxylase (GAD65)and auto antibodies to the tyrosine phosphatases, 1A-2A and 1A- 2B.

↓ **Idiopathic:** This is of no known etiology. Some of these patients have permanent insulinopenia and are prone to ketoacidosis, but have no evidence of auto immunity. Many races of African and Asian origin fall into this group.

(B) Type 2 or maturity (or) adult onset dm (or) insulin resistace syndrome (or) metabolic syndrome

Earlier known as non-insulin dependent diabetes mellitus (NIDDM) or adult-onset diabetes. This is the most common form of diabetes, and is strongly associated with genetic tendency and obesity. The body produces normal or even high levels of insulin, but certain factors make its utilization ineffective ("insulin resistance"). Sedentary lifestyle, unhealthy dietary patterns, and   the consequent obesity are common causes.

This is characterized by variable insulin secretion that may be due to an inadequate β-cell function of the pancreas. Etiological factors includes heredity , abnormality in gluco receptors of β-cells so that they respond at higher glucose concentration, reduced sensitivity of peripheral tissues to insulin, reduction in the no. of insulin receptors and down regulation, excess of hyperglycemic hormones (glucagon), cardio vascular disorders etc.

c) Gestational diabetes mellitus or pregnancy-induced diabetes. Gestational diabetes is usually identified during the second trimester of pregnancy. In this condition, the pregnancy hormones inhibit the action of insulin due to which the glucose produced in the body is not utilised for providing energy. The glucose level in the body increases leading to hyperglycaemia and the body tissues are deprived of energy. High blood sugar can damage the health of the fetus. Some of the complications for the baby include premature delivery, respiratory problems, congestive heart failure and decreased ability to tolerate labor.

d) Secondary diabetes mellitus, caused by genetic conditions, pancreatic diseases (e.g. inflammation, surgery or malignancy of the pancreas, etc.), drugs (e.g. steroids like prednisolone, pentamidine, excess thyroid hormone, etc.) or other medical conditions (acromegaly, Cushing syndrome, pheochromocytoma, hyperthyroidism, congenital rubella, etc). Medications such as thiazide diuretics or oral contraceptives can precipitate diabetes in a person predisposed to get it later.

(1.1.3.2) Sign and symptoms

↓ Type (I) diabetes

A primary symptom is in the form of nausea and vomiting. In later stage, which leads to diabetic ketoacidosis, a state of metabolic deregulation characterized by the smell of acetone, the body starts breaking down the muscle tissue and fat for producing energy hence, causing fast weight loss. Dehydrations is also usually observed due to electrolyte disturbance. In advanced stages, coma and death is witnessed.

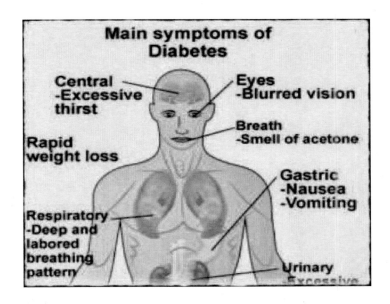

Figure 1.1.3.2 a

↓ Type(II) diabetes

Increase fatigue,Excessive thirst (Polydipsia,)Excessive urination, (Polyuria) Excessive eating, (polyphagia).Poor wound healing Infections, Blurry vision,Altered mental status, Agitation, unexplained irritability, inattention, extreme lethargy, or confusion can all be signs of very high blood sugar, ketoacidosis, hyperosmolar, nonketonic syndrome hyperglycemia, or hypoglycemia. (Leon.et al.,2014).

Pancreas:

The pancreas is called a retroperitoneal organ. That means it lies within the peritoneal cavity but outside (behind) the visceral peritoneum or membrane.

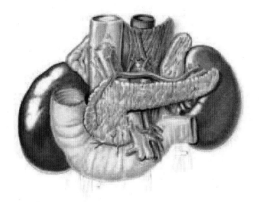

Figure 2a

Anatomy and pathophysiology of pancreas:

Anatomy:

The pancreas is located in the middle to upper abdominal cavity, towards the back or posterior. It is about 12 inches long and tapers from right to left.

the pancreas in terms of its head and tail. As for the front surface of the pancreas, it rests mostly against the back (posterior) wall of the stomach.

Endocrine and exocrine functions coexist in the pancreas. By definition, endocrine organs secrete hormones directly into the bloodstream, whereas exocrine organs secrete hormones directly into the cavity (lumen) of another organ.

The exocrine pancreas comprises 99% of pancreatic tissue. It secretes digestive juices into the duct system that carry them on into the cavity of the duodenum

Pathophysiology:

The endocrine pancreas, on the other hand, secretes hormones (insulin, glucagon, and somatostatin) directly into the bloodstream.

The major stimulation of the pancreas is primarily parasympathetic (originating in the brain stem), through the vagus nerve, and promotes secretion of digestive juices. Parasympathetic stimulation to the pancreas occurs in response to the digestive processes of the stomach.

Inhibition of pancreatic secretion of digestive juices is controlled by triggers and nerves outside of the central nervous system -- the sympathetic nervous system. Specifically, when acid chyme enters the duodenum, along with partially digested fats, proteins, and carbohydrates, enteroendocrine cells in the duodenum and small intestine release cholecystokinin (CCK) and secretin. Secretin decreases gastric secretion and CCK inhibits gastric emptying.

These two enzymes circulate into the bloodstream. In addition, they stimulate further secretion of pancreatic enzymes and sodium bicarbonate into the small intestine, thus further raising the pH in the duodenum.

Insulin (Birkeland et al., 2011) Both type 1 and type 2 diabetes share one central feature: elevated blood sugar (glucose) levels due to absolute or relative insufficiencies of insulin, a hormone produced by the pancreas. Insulin is a key regulator of the body's metabolism. It works in the following way:

- During and immediately after a meal, digestion breaks carbohydrates down into sugar molecules (of which glucose is one) and proteins into amino acids.
- Right after the meal, glucose and amino acids are absorbed directly into the bloodstream, and blood glucose levels rise sharply. (Glucose levels after a meal are called *postprandial* levels.)

- The rise in blood glucose levels signals important cells in the pancreas, called *beta cells*, to secrete insulin, which pours into the bloodstream. Within 20 minutes after a meal insulin rises to its peak level.
- Insulin enables glucose to enter cells in the body, particularly muscle and liver cells. Here, insulin and other hormones direct whether glucose will be burned for energy or stored for future use.

- When insulin levels are high, the liver stops producing glucose and stores it in other forms until the body needs it again.
- As blood glucose levels reach their peak, the pancreas reduces the production of insulin.
- About 2 - 4 hours after a meal both blood glucose and insulin are at low levels, with insulin being slightly higher. The blood glucose levels are then referred to as *fasting*
- The pancreas is located behind the liver and stomach. In addition to secreting digestive enzymes, the pancreas secretes the hormones insulin and glucagon into the bloodstream. The release of insulin into the blood lowers the level of blood glucose (simple sugars from food) by enhancing glucose to enter the body cells, where it is metabolized. If blood glucose levels get too low, the pancreas secretes glucagon to stimulate the release of glucose from the liver.

Table 2.2.1.5 Types of insulin (Katzung et al 2009)

Types	Appearance	Added protein	Onset (hr)	Duration	ROUTE	CHANGES IN AMINO ACID SEQUENCES
Rapid acting analogs						
Lispro	Clear	None	5-15 min.	4-6	s.c.	Proline at position B 28 has been moved to B29 and lysine B29 and moved to B28.
Aspart	Clear	None	0.25	3-5	s.c.	Proline at position B 28 has been moved to B29 and lysine B29 and moved to B28.
Glulisine	Clear	None	-	1-2.5	s.c.	Lysine at B3 and glutamic acid lysine at B29.
Intermediate						
NPH	Cloudy	Protamine	1-2hrs.	10-18hrs.	s.c.	---------
Lente	Cloudy	None	1-2	18-24	s.c.	----------
Long acting						
Ultralente	Cloudy	None	4-6	20-36	s.c.	----------
Protamine	Cloudy	Protamine	4-6	24-36	s.c.	----------

Glargine	Clear	None	2-5	18-24	s.c.	2 Arginine on B chain and glycine for aspargine at A21.
Determir	Clear	None	1-2	6-24	s.c.	Attached to the B29 lysine.
Short acting Regular human (Humulin,N ovolin)	Clear		30-60min.	6-10	i.v.	-----------

Newer insulin delivery devices (Tripathi et al.,2013)

A number of innovations have been made to improve ease and accuracy of insulin administration as well as to achieve tight glycaemia control.

These are:

- **Insulin syringes:** Prefilled disposable syringes contain specific types or mixture of regular and modified insulin.
- **Pen devices:** Fountain pen like use insulin cartridges for s.c. injection through a needle. Preset amounts (in 2U increments) are propelled by pushing a plunger convenient in carrying and injecting.
- **Inhaled insulin:** An inhaled human insulin preparation was marketed in Europe and the U.S.A, but withdrawn due to risk of pulmonary fibrosis and other complications. The fine powder delivered through a nebulizer controlled meal time glycaemia,but was not suitable for round the clock basal effect. Attempts are being made to overcome the shortcomings.

Insulin Pumps: Portable insulin devices connected to a sub cutaneous placed cannula provide continuous subcutaneous insulin infusion (CS II).only regular insulin or a fast acting insulin analogue is used. The pump can be programmed to deliver insulin at a low basal rate (approx.1U/hr) and premeal boluses (4-15 times the basal rate) to control post- prandial glycaemia. Though theoretically more appealing, no definite advantage of CS II over multidose S.C. injection has been demonstrated. Moreover, cost, strict adherence to diet, exercise ,care of device and cannula, risk of pump failure, site injection are to demanding on the patient. The CSII may be appropriate for selected type 2 DM cases only.

Implantable pumps: Consist of an electromechanical mechanism which regulates insulin delivery from from a percutaneously refillable reservoir. Mechanical pumps, propellant driven and osmotic pumps have been utilized. Other routes of insulin delivery: Intraperitoneal, oral (by complexing insulin into liposomes or coating it with impermeable polymer) and rectal routes are being tried.

These have the advantage of providing higher concentrations in the portal circulation, which is more physiological.

Metabolic regulation of insulin

The stimulation of insulin secretion by glucose requires several steps.

- Penetration of glucose into beta cells, by Glut2 carriers, independently of the presence of insulin.
- Phosphorylation of glucose by glucokinase, then its metabolisation with synthesis of ATP whose intracellular concentration increases. This increase in ATP induces the closing of ATP-dependant potassium channels and the cessation of potassium exit, with as a consequence depolarization and opening of the voltage-dependant calcium channels. The entry of calcium elicits the activation of A2 and C phospholipases and the secretion of insulin.

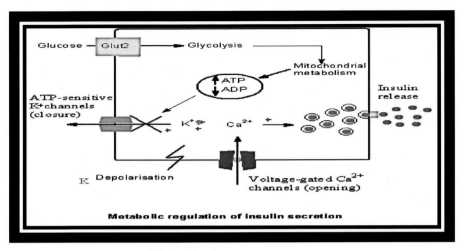

Figure 2 b

Mechanism of Insulin:

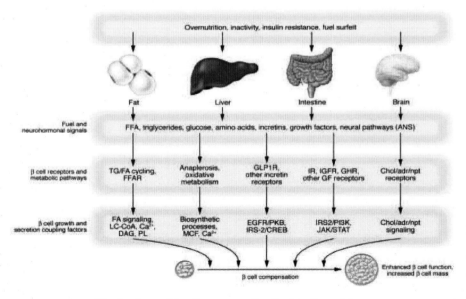

Mechanisms of β cell compensation for insulin resistance.

Figure 2 c

Normally islet β cells respond to insulin resistance by increased secretion through the processes of compensation. These include an expansion of β cell mass, increased insulin biosynthesis, and enhanced nutrient secretion coupling processes with increased sensitivity to glucose, FFAs, and GLP-1 stimuli. Enhanced glucose utilization, glucose oxidation, anaplerosis/cataplerosis, and TG/FFA cycling result in increased production of coupling signals necessary for insulin exocytose. For expansion of β cell mass, roles are evident for increased activity of growth factor signaling pathways, postprandial glucose, and GLP-1 signaling that promote β cell proliferation and neogenesis and prevent apoptosis. Furthermore, signaling for growth may occur in response to FFAs, via the FFA receptors (FFAR) and via lipid signaling molecules derived from TG/FFA cycling. adr, adrenergic; ANS, autonomic nervous system; chol, cholinergic; CREB, cAMP response element–binding protein; DAG, diacylglycerol; GF, growth factor; GLP1R, GLP-1 receptor; GHR, growth hormone receptor; IGFR, insulin-like growth factor receptor; IR, insulin receptor, IRS-2, insulin receptor substrate 2; MCF, metabolic coupling factors; neuropeptide; PKB, phosphokinase B; phospholipids.

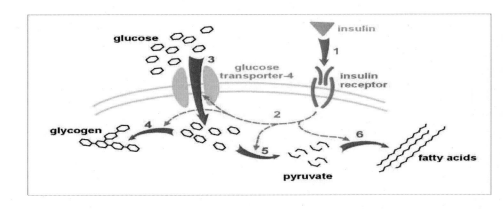

Effect of insulin on glucose uptake and metabolism

Figure 2 d

(1) Insulin binds to its receptor (2) on the cell membrane which in turn starts many protein activation cascades (3). These include: translocation of Glut-4 transporter to the plasma membrane and influx of glucose (4), glycogen synthesis (5), glycolysis (6) and fatty acid synthesis.

Causes of diabetes

Autoimmune Response

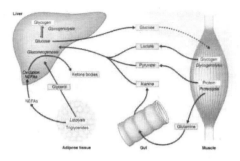

Figure 2 e

Type i diabetes is considered a progressive *autoimmune* disease, in which the beta cells that produce insulin are slowly destroyed by the body's own immune system. It is unknown what first starts this process. Evidence suggests that both a genetic predisposition and environmental factors, such as a viral infection, are involved.

Type 1 Diabetes is autoimmune disease that affects 0.3% on average. it is result of destruction of beta cells due to aggressive nature of cells present in the body. some of the diabetes occurs in Type 1 may be genetic, poor diet (malnutrition) and environment (virus affecting pancreas).Secondary inmost of cases diabetes occurs because there is abnormal secretion of some hormones in blood which act as antagonists to insulin. **Example** Adrenocortical hormone, Adrenaline hormone and Thyroid hormone.

Type ii Diabetes

Type 2 Diabetes is also called non insulin-dependent diabetes mellitus (NIDDM) or adult-onset diabetes.

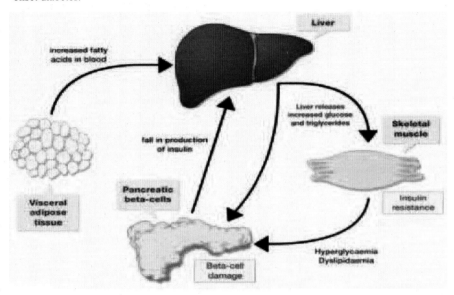

(a) Genetic Factors   **Figure 2 f**

Researchers have found at least 18 genetic locations, labeled IDDM1 - IDDM18, which are related to type 1 diabetes.Most people who develop type 1 diabetes do not have a family history of the disease. The odds of inheriting the disease are only 10% if a first-degree relative has diabetes and, even in identical twins, one twin has only a 33% chance of having type 1 diabetes if the other twin has it. Children are more likely to inherit the disease from a father with type 1 diabetes than from a mother with the disorder.Genetic factors cannot fully explain the development of diabetes. For the past several decades, the number of new cases of type 1 diabetes has been increasing each year worldwide.

(b)Viruses

Some research suggests that viral infections may trigger the disease in genetically susceptible individuals.Among the viruses under scrutiny are *enteric* viruses, which attack the intestinal tract. Coxsackie viruses are a family of enteric viruses of particular interest. Epidemics of Coxsackie virus, as well as mumps and congenital rubella, have been associated with type 1 diabetes.

Complications (Colledge et al., 2010)

Type 1 diabetes increases the risk for many serious health complications. However, during the past several decades, the rate of serious complications among people with diabetes has been decreasing, and more patients are living longer and healthier lives. There are two important approaches to preventing complications from type 1 diabetes:

- ☐ Good control of blood glucose and keeping glycosylated hemoglobin (A1C) levels below or around 7%. This approach can help prevent complications due to vascular (blood vessel) abnormalities and nerve damage (neuropathy) that can cause major damage to organs, including the eyes, kidneys, and heart.
- ☐ Managing risk factors for heart disease. Blood glucose control helps the heart, but it is also very important that people with diabetes control blood pressure, cholesterol levels, and other factors associated with heart disease.

Diabetic Ketoacidosis

Diabetic ketoacidosis (DKA) is a life-threatening complication caused by a complete (or almost complete) lack of insulin. In DKA, the body produces abnormally high levels of blood acids called ketones. Ketones are by products of fat breakdown that build up in the blood and appear in the urine.

They are produced when the body burns fat instead of glucose for energy. The buildup of ketones in the body is called ketoacidosis. Extreme stages of diabetic ketoacidosis can lead to coma and death.

For some people, DKA may be the first sign that someone has diabetes. In type 1 diabetes, it usually occurs when a patient is not compliant with insulin therapy or intentionally reduces insulin doses in order to lose weight.

It can also be triggered by a severe illness or infection.

Diabetic Ketoacidosis

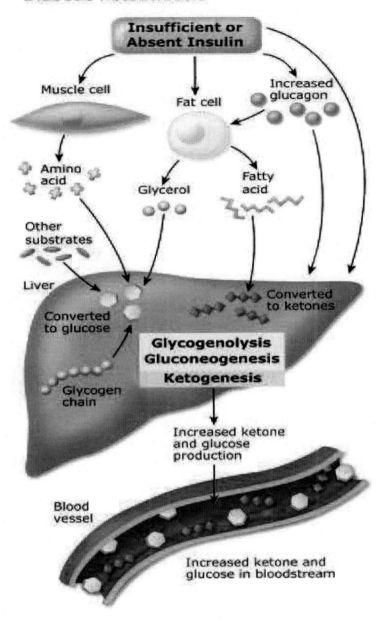

Figure 2 g.

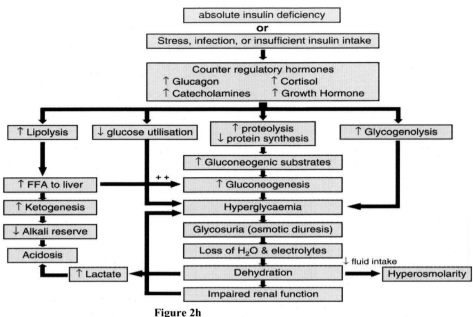

Figure 2h

Symptoms and complications include:

- Thirst and dry mouth,Frequent urination,Fatigue,Dry warm skin,Nausea and vomiting and stomach pain, Confusion and decreased consciousness coma, brain damage, or death.
- Other serious complications from DKA include aspiration pneumonia and adult respiratory distress syndrome.

Life-saving treatment uses rapid replacement of fluids with a salt (saline) solution followed by low-dose insulin and potassium replacement.Ketoacidosis is a serious condition of glucose build-up in the blood and urine. A simple urine test can determine if high ketone levels are present.

❖ **Hyperglycemic Hyperosmolar Nonketonic Syndrome (HHNS)**

Hyperglycemic hyperosmolar nonketonic syndrome (HHNS) is a serious complication of diabetes that involves a cycle of increasing blood sugar levels and dehydration, without ketones. HHNS usually occurs with type 2 diabetes, but it can also occur with type 1 diabetes. It is often triggered by a serious infection or another severe illness, or by medications that lower glucose tolerance or increase fluid loss (especially in people who are not drinking enough fluids).

Symptoms of HHNS include high blood sugar levels, dry mouth, extreme thirst, dry skin, and high fever. HHNS can lead to loss of consciousness, seizures, coma, and death.

❖ Hypoglycemia:

Tight blood sugar (glucose) control increases the risk of low blood sugar (hypoglycemia). Hypoglycemia occurs if blood glucose levels fall below normal. It is generally defined as a blood sugar below 70 mg/dl, although this level may not necessarily cause symptoms in all patients. Insufficient intake of food and excess exercise or alcohol intake may cause hypoglycemia. Usually the condition is manageable, but, occasionally, it can be severe or even life threatening, particularly if the patient fails to recognize the symptoms, especially while continuing to take insulin or other hypoglycemic drugs. Beta-blocking medications, which are often prescribed for high blood pressure and heart disease, can mask symptoms of hypoglycemia.

These are 2 types   **(1) Micro vascular**   **(2) Macro vascular**

(1) Micro vascular (Colledge et al., 2010)

Kidney Damage (Nephropathy) Kidney disease (nephropathy) is a very serious complication of diabetes. With this condition, the tiny filters in the kidney (called glomerul) become damaged and leak protein into the urine. Over time this can lead to kidney failure. Urine tests showing microalbuminuria (small amounts of protein in the urine) are important markers for kidney damage.

Diabetic nephropathy is the leading cause of end-stage renal disease (ESRD). Patients with ESRD have 13 times the risk of death compared to other patients with type 1 diabetes. If the kidneys fail, dialysis or transplantation is required. Symptoms of kidney failure may include

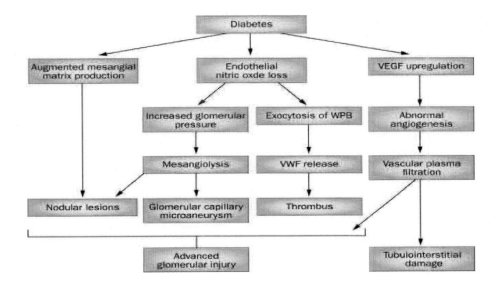

Figure 2 i

Swelling in the feet and ankles, itching, fatigue, and pale skin color. The outlook of end-stage renal disease has greatly improved during the last four decades for patients with type 1 diabetes, and fewer people with type 1 diabetes are developing ESRD.

(b) Neuropathy

Diabetes reduces or distorts nerve function, causing a condition called neuropathy. Neuropathy refers to a group of disorders that affect nerves. The two main types of neuropathy are:

☐ *Peripheral*   (affects nerves in the toes, feet, legs, hand, and arms)

☐ *Autonomic* (affects nerves that help regulate digestive, bowel, bladder, heart, and sexual function)

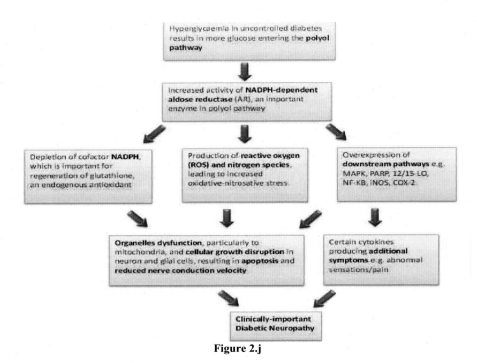

Figure 2.j

Peripheral neuropathy particularly affects sensation. It is a common complication for nearly half of people who have lived with type 1 or type 2 diabetes for more than 25 years. The most serious consequences of neuropathy occur in the legs and feet and pose a risk for ulcers and, in unusually severe cases, amputation. Peripheral neuropathy usually starts in the fingers and toes and moves up to the arms and legs (called a stocking-glove distribution). Symptoms include:

☐ Tingling,Weakness,Burning sensations ,Loss of the sense of warm or cold,Numbness (if the nerves are severely damaged, the patient may be unaware that a blister or minor wound has become infected),Deep pain.

Autonomic neuropathy can cause:

☐ Digestive problems (such as constipation, diarrhea, nausea, and vomiting)

☐ Bladder infections and incontinence

☐ Erectile dysfunction

☐ Heart problems. Neuropathy may mask angina, the warning chest pain for heart disease and heart attack. Patients with diabetes should be aware of other warning signs of a heart attack, including sudden fatigue, sweating, shortness of breath, nausea, and vomiting.

☐ Rapid heart rates

☐ Lightheadedness when standing up (orthostatic hypotension)

☐ Diabetic gastro paresis is a type of neuropathy that affects the digestive track. It is triggered by high blood sugar, which over time can damage the vagus nerve. The result of this damage is that the digestive system takes too long at time to move and empty food. Undigested food and the delay in stomach emptying can cause blood glucose levels to rise, and make diabetes more difficult to control. Symptoms of gastro paresis include heartburn, nausea, abdominal bloating, feeling full after eating only a small amount of food, and vomiting of undigested food several hours after a meal.

☐ Blood sugar control is an essential component in the treatment for neuropathy. Studies show that tight control of blood glucose levels delays the onset and slows progression of neuropathy. Heart disease risk factors may increase the likelihood of developing neuropathy. Lowering triglycerides, losing weight, reducing blood pressure, and quitting smoking may help prevent the onset of neuropathy.

(b) Foot Ulcers and Amputations

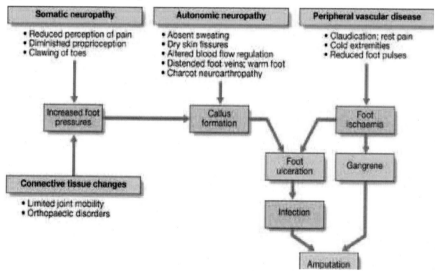

☐ About 15% of patients with diabetes have serious foot problems. They are the leading cause of hospitalizations for these patients. The consequences of both poor circulation and peripheral neuropathy make this a common and serious problem for all patients with diabetes. Diabetes is responsible for more than half of all lower limb amputations performed in the U.S. Most amputations start with foot ulcers.

- People with diabetes who are overweight, smokers, and have a long history of diabetes tend to be at most risk. People who have the disease for more than 20 years and are insulin-dependent are at the highest risk. Related conditions that put people at risk include peripheral neuropathy, peripheral artery disease, foot deformities, and a history of ulcers.

- Foot ulcers usually develop from infections, such as those resulting from blood vessel injury. Numbness from nerve damage, which is common in diabetes, compounds the danger since the patient may not be aware of injuries. About one-third of foot ulcers occur on the big toe.

- *Charcot Foot.* Charcot foot or Charcot joint (medically referred to as neuropathic arthropathy) is a degenerative condition that affects the bones and joints in the feet. It is associated with the nerve damage that occurs with neuropathy. Early changes appear similar to an infection, with the foot becoming swollen, red, and warm. Gradually, the affected foot can become deformed. The bones may crack, splinter, and erode, and the joints may shift, change shape, and become unstable. It typically develops in people who have neuropathy to the extent that they cannot feel sensation in the foot and are not aware of an existing injury. Instead of resting an injured foot or seeking medical help, the patient often continues normal activity, causing further damage.

(d) Retinopathy and Eye Complications

- Diabetes accounts for thousands of new cases of blindness annually and is the leading cause of new cases of blindness in adults ages 20 - 74. The most common eye disorder in diabetes is retinopathy. People with diabetes are also at higher risk for developing cataracts and certain types of glaucoma.

Diabetic Retinopathy

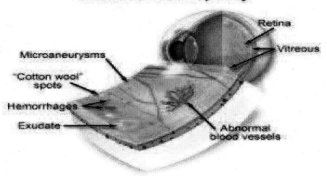

Figure 2 k

☐ Retinopathy is a condition in which the retina becomes damaged. It generally occurs in one or two phases:

☐ The early and more common type of this disorder is called *non proliferative or background retinopathy*. The blood vessels in the retina are abnormally weakened. They rupture and leak, and waxy areas may form. If these processes affect the central portion of the retina, swelling may occur, causing reduced or blurred vision.

☐ If the capillaries become blocked and blood flow is cut off, soft, "woolly" areas may develop in the retina's nerve layer. These woolly areas may signal the development of *proliferative retinopathy*. In this more severe condition, new abnormal blood vessels form and grow on the surface of the retina. They may spread into the cavity of the eye or bleed into the back of the eye. Major hemorrhage or retinal detachment can result, causing severe visual loss or blindness. The sensation of seeing flashing lights may indicate retinal detachment.

☐ Diabetes mellitus comes from the Greek word "diabainein" meaning "to pass through," and the Latin word "mellitus" meaning "sweetened with honey." Put the two words together and you have "to pass through sweetened with honey."

(2) Macro vascular:

❖ **Heart Disease and Stroke**

Patients with type 1 diabetes are 10 times more at risk for heart disease than healthy patients. Heart attacks account for 60% of deaths in patients with diabetes, while strokes account for 25% of such deaths. Diabetes affects the heart in many ways:

☐ Both type 1 and 2 diabetes accelerate the progression of atherosclerosis (hardening of the arteries). Diabetes is often associated with low HDL ("good" cholesterol) and high triglycerides. This can lead to coronary artery disease, heart attack, or stroke.

☐ In type 1 diabetes, high blood pressure (hypertension) usually develops if the kidneys become damaged. High blood pressure is another major cause of heart attack, stroke, and heart failure. Children with diabetes are also at risk for hypertension.

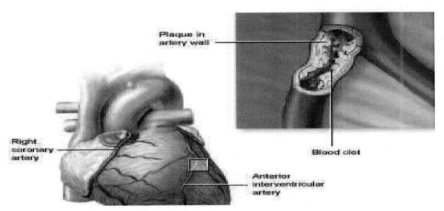

☐ Impaired nerve function (neuropathy) associated with diabetes also causes heart abnormalities.

Atherosclerosis is a disease of the arteries in which fatty material is deposited in the vessel wall, resulting in narrowing and eventual impairment of blood flow. Severely restricted blood flow in the arteries to the heart muscle leads to symptoms such as chest pain. Atherosclerosis shows no symptoms until a complication occurs.

29

2.2.1.11 CLASSIFICATION (Katzung et al.,2009,Tripathi et al.,2013. FDA 2010-2014).

DRUG	M.O.A	ADVERSE EFFECT	DOSE	DURATION OF ACTION (hours)	CLINICAL APPLICATION	A1C DECREASE %	FDA APPROVAL
Sulfonylurea *First Generation* Tolbutamide Chlorpropamide,Tolazamide, *Second Generation* Glibenclamide, Glipizide, Gliclazide, Gliquidone,	Stimulating insulin release by pancreatic β cells by inhibiting the KATP.	Hypoglycaemia, weight gain,	0.5-2g in divided doses 0.1-0.5 g as single dose. 0.001-0.004 g 12-240.005-0.03 g (0.02 g in glucotrol XL)	6-12 Upto 60 18-24 hrs. 16-24 hrs.	Type2 diabetes 10-24	1-2	2012

Biguanides Metformin	Acts on liver to cause decrease in insulin resistance.	Anorexia ,diarrhea,nausea . Vitamin B12 deficiency.	1.5-3	Less than 4 hours	Type2 diabetes	1.5-2.0	2010

Thiazolidinedi ones Pioglitazone Rosiglitazone.	Decrease blood glucose levels,by reducing insulin resistace in adipose tissue,mus cle,and liver.increa se insulin sensitivity.	Weight gain,mild or moderate edema,headach, hepatotoxicity,	15-45 mg once daily.	2 hrs.	Type 2	1.5-2.0	2010 2010 and suspended Due to cardiovasc ular risk.
Meglitinides /Phenylalanin e analogues Repaglinide,N atiglinide	Activate insulin receptors.	Low risk of hypoglycaemia.	0.25-4 mg before meals.	4-5	Tpe 1 and Type 2 diabetes.	0.5-1.0	2010
α – Glycosidase inhibitors Acarbose	Reduces glucose absorbance by acting on small intestine to cause decrease in production of enzyme needed to carbohydra tes.	Nausea,vomitin g,and anorexia.diarrho ea,loose stool.	25-100mg before meal.	20-50 min.	Type 2	0.5-1.0	2010

Sodium– glucose cotransport-2 Canagliflozin Dapaglliflozin	Lower the renal glucose threshold resulting in increase amount of glucose being excreted.	Urinary tact infection.	100mg and 300 mg	30 min.	Type 2	 0.90	2013 2014
New antidiabetic(in cretin based drugs) drugs. Byetta(Exenati de) GLP-1. Januvia(Sitagli ptin) (DPP-4)	Substance secreted by the body that stimulates insulin secretion. Drug inhibit the destruction of GLP-1 blood levels so will extended the action of GLP-1and will increase the insulin secretion.	Appetite Weight gain,hypoglycae mia.s	60 mint.before meal. 100 mg once daily	2-10 hrs 12 hrs.	Type 2 Type 2	0.5-1.0 0.5-1.0 0.7	 2010

Animal models in experimental diabetes mellitus and studies for antidiabetic activity

There are many advantages of using animal models in research work on diabetes as various aspects of the disease like the etiology, its multifactorial genetics, pathogenesis of the disease and its complications can be explicitly understood. Secondly, it also helps in the development and evaluation of newer agents for the treatment of diabetes (Chattopadhyay et al., 1997)

Induction of diabetes in animals can be carried out by various ways -by using different chemical diabetogens (Dunn et al, 1943a and Rerup, 1970) surgically by partial pancreatectomy (Bonner-Weir et al, 1983), by viral induction (Craighead et al., 1968 and Hayashi et al., 1974) and genetic manipulation by selective breeding (Karasik et al., 1986). Induction of diabetes by various chemical diabetogens is also dependant on the species, the strain, sex and the diet of the animal.

Alloxan:

Chemically alloxan is 2, 4, 5,6,tetra-oxo-hexahydropyrimidine. Alloxan was one of the most widely used experimental diabetes model. It is freely soluble in water and slightly acidic with a pKa of 6.63 (Labes et al., 1930). On standing at room temperature it decomposes to alloxantin, oxalate, urea, carbon dioxide and other chemical substances, but at low pH 3, the aqueous solution of alloxan is fairly stable. Alloxan acts as a diabetogen in rats, mice, rabbits, dogs, hamster, sheep and monkey but guinea pigs are Sresistant to alloxan induced diabetes (Rerup, 1970 and Johnson, 1950).

Neonates though very young animals, are resistant to the diabetogenic effect of alloxan (Creutzfeldt et al., 1949). Alloxan can be administered virtually through all routes, i.e, i.v. (Bailey et al., 1943), i.m. (Dunn et al., 1943), i.p. (Gomori et al., 1943), s.c. (Dunn et al., 1943b) and also by oral route. Owing to its short half life (less than 1 min) it is best administered by infusion in the pancreatic artery. The exact mechanism of β-cell destruction is not clear but several hypothesis have been put forward (Rerup, 1970).

In normal non-fasted animals the blood glucose level after alloxan injection fluctuates in the triphasic pattern. There is early marked hyperglycemia of s hort duration followed by hypoglycemia of short duration, followed by hyperglycemia of long duration. Permanent diabetes produced by alloxan was found to be associated with ketoacidosis in dogs and cats and required insulin treatment for survival, whereas with rats and mice, spontaneous remission was reported (Lazarow, 1952; Rerup, 1968).

Streptozotocin:

Streptozotocin is a broad spectrum antibiotic isolated from *Streptomyces achromogenes* in 1959 (Herr et al., 1959-1960). Earlier this compound was reported to have anticancer activity (Evans et al., 1965; Arison et al., 1967) and its diabetic property was first reported by Rakieten and co-workers (Schein et al., 1968). Chemically, STZ is 1-methyl-1-nitrosourea linked to position C_2 pg D-glucose. It is freely soluble in water, unstable at room temperature and has to be stored below 20ºC. In solution form at room temperature and at neutral pH it decomposes with the formation of gas. Its stability in solution is optimum at pH 4 and low temperatures. The biological half life was found to be 5 min in mice (Schein et al., 1968).

Lithium:

Lithium salts are widely used in the treatment of manic-depressive psychosis and allied diseases. Its exact mechanism of action as a mood stabilizing agent is not yet clearly known and number of postulations have been forwarded. It has been reported that lithium has a significant effects on endocrine pancreas as well (Craig et al., 1977 and Johnson, 1977). It has been shown to inhibit glucose stimulated insulin release in rats after either in vitro or in vivo administration (Anderson et al.,1978) leading to glucose intolerance. Lithium stimulates the alpha adrenoceptors leading to increased plasma glucose levels and inhibits the release of insulin from the pancreatic islet cells (Fontela et al., 1986 and Fontela et al., 1990). Intravenous infusion of lithium at a dose of 4m eq/kg into the jugular vein of anaesthetized rats produced an elevation of blood glucose levels within 30 min to 7-8 n mol/L and by 2 hrs, the animals became normoglycemic. This hyperglycemic effect of lithium may be due to its effect on the sympatho-adrenal function, both directly and indirectly, leading to decreased release of insulin from beta cells of the pancreas (Bhattacharya, 1964).

REVIEW OF LITERATURE OF PLANT PROFILE

Botanical name: *Spondias pinnata* (Linn. f.) Kurz.

Family: Anacandiaceae

Vernicular names:

English	Hog plum
Hindi	Amara, Ambodha
Punjabi	Ambara
Sanskrit	Amrata
Urdu	Jangali Aam

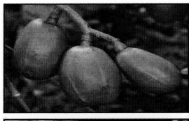
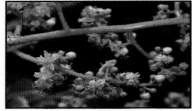

Fig.2.13. Spondias pinnata.

Chemical Constituents:

- Phytochemical studies have yielded flavonoids, tannins, saponins and terpenoids.

- Essential oil from the pulp yielded carboxylic acids and esters, alcohols, aromatic hydrocarbons. Fruits yield ß-amyrin, oeanolic acid, glycine, cystine, serine, alanine, and leucine. Aerial parts yield lignoceric acid, ß-sitosterol and its glucoside.(Kirtikar et al.,1935).

  Medicinal properties: (Kirtikar et al.,1935).

The fruits are eaten as a vegetable when green and as a fruit when ripe. They are used for flavoring. The flowers are sour and used in curry as a flavoring and also eaten raw as well as the local people make chutney, jam and pickle. Fruits are very nutritious and rich in vitamin A, minerals and iron content. The bark is useful in dysentery and diarrhea and is also prevent vomiting. The root is considered useful in regulating menstruation. The plant is reported to have anti-tubercular properties. The leaves are aromatic, acidic and astringent

Pharmacological Review:

❖ **Hypoglycaemic activity**

Mondal et al., (2009) evaluated for hypoglycemic activity on adult Wistar albino rats at dose levels of 300 mg/kg p.o. each using normoglycaemic, glucose loaded and alloxan induced for 14 days. Glibenclamide (2.5 mg/kg) was used as reference standard for activity comparison. Among the tested extracts, the methanol extract was found to produce promising results that is comparable to that of the reference standard glibenclamide. The preliminary phytochemical examination of the methanol extract revealed presence of flavonoids, tannins, saponins and terpenoids. The present work justifies the use of the bark in the folklore treatment in diabetes.

Hepatoprotective activity:

Hazra et al., (2013) evaluated the hepatoprotective activity of *Spondias pinnata* with 70% methanol extract *spondias pinnata* (SPME) on iron overload induced liver injury. Iron overload was induced by intraperitoneal administration of iron -dextran into mice. Results were demonstrated the hepatoprotective efficiency of SPME in iron intoxicated mice, hence possibly useful as iron chelating drug for iron overload diseases.

❖ *In vitro* **anticancer activity:**

Ghate et al., (2013) investigated on *Spondias pinnata* bark on human lung and breast carcinoma with 70 % methanolic extract of *Spondias pinnata* bark (SPME) in promoting apoptosis in human lung adenocarcinoma cell line (A549) and human breast adenocarcinoma cell line (MCF-7).

❖ **Antidiarrheal activity:**

Panda et al., (2012) Studied antibacterial activity using agar well diffusion (concentration 100mg/ml) against eight phathogenic bacteria responsible for diarrheal diseases.

❖ **Antioxidant activity:**

Chalise et al., (2010) Studied for the antioxidant activity and total polyphenol content (TPC), which results to beneficial health effects due to their antioxidant activity and TPC.

❖ **Diuretic and laxative activity:**

Mondal et al., (2009) Studied diuretic and laxative activity of different bark extracts of *Spondias pinnata* in wistar albino rat. The chloroform and methanol extracts produced significant diuretic and laxative activity.

❖ **Antioxidant and free radical scavenging activity:**

Hazra. et al., (2008) Evaluated antioxidant activities of spondias pinnata stem bark extract which provided evidence that 70% methanol extract of *spondias pinnata* stem bark is a potential source of natural antioxidant.

Phytochemical Review:

Tandon et al., (1976) studied the chemical constituents of *Spondias pinnata*. Aerial parts of the plant was reported to contain 24-methylene-cycloartanone, stigma-4en-3-one, β-sitosterol, lignoceric acid and β-sitosterol β-D-glucoside.

Ongoing research work in the area of the proposal:

⬥ Unakal et al.,(2014) evaluated antidiabetic activity of Amaranthus dubiousethanolic leaf extract on alloxan induced diabetic mice. Intraperitoneal administration of alloxan monohydrate (200mg/kg body weight) for 45 days. leaf extract exhibited antidiabetic activity by improving the peripheral utilization of glucose by altering the impaired liver glycolysis and by limiting its gluconeogenic formation similar to insulin. This effect may be due to the presence of alkaloids, flavanoids,galloatnoids, and other constituents present in the leaf which could act by synergistically in improving the activity of glycolytic and gluconeogenic enzymes.

⬥ Tabassum et al.,(2014) investigated the pharmacological study on antinociceptive and antihyperglycemic effects of Allium cepa leaves in Swiss albino mice 10 ml/kg body weight) . Each mouse was weighed and doses adjusted accordingly prior to administration of vehicle, standard drug, and test samples. All substances were orally administered for 3 days. t-test was carried out for statistical comparison. Statistical significance was considered to be indicated by a p value < 0.05.

❖ Li..,et al.,(2014) evaluated antidiabetic effect of flavonoids from Malus toringoides (Rehd.) Hughes leaves in diabetic mice and rats.and 45 mg/kg . Both mice and rats were fasted for 5 h before administration and the blood glucose (BG) levels were tested 1 h after treatment. STZ-induced rats, glycosylated hemoglobin (Hb1Ac), serum insulin and c-peptide, hepatic glycogen, superoxide dismutase (SOD) activity and malondialdehyde (MDA) levels in liver were assessed on the fourth day after BG level detection. BG levels were significantly reduced (P<0.05). Significant decrease (P<0.05) in Hb1Ac level was observed in ESF-treated rats compared with diabetic rats. Significant increase (P<0.05) in serum insulin and c-peptide were detected in ESF-treated rats. The treatment also significantly (P<0.05) elevated SOD activity and reduced MDA level in the liver of diabetic rats.

- Karuppusamy et al., (2013) evaluated the effect of methanolic extract of the bark of *Ficus amplissim* on streptozotocin-induced diabetic rats. Oral administration of bark at the doses of 50mg/kg, 100mg/kg and150mg/Kg was studied in normal, glucose-loaded and STZ—induced dose 55mg/kg for 21 days. The anti-diabetic effect of was compared with glibenclamide.

- Kamboj et al.,(2013) evaluation of Antidiabetic Activity of Hydroalcoholic extract of Cestrum nocturnum Leaves in Streptozotocin-Induced Diabetic Rats. Hyperglyc emia was induced by injecting streptozotocin at a dose of 150 mg/kg i.p for 15 days. Phytochemical analysis of Cestrum nocturnum leaves showed the presence of flavonoids, tannins, saponins, sterols, and triterpenoids. a significant reduction in blood glucose levels in diabetic rats. The body weight of diabetic animals was also improved after daily administration of extracts.

- N et al.,(2013) investigated antidiabetic and antihyperlipidemic activity of Piper longum root aqueous extract in STZ induced diabetic rats. Diabetes was induced in male Wister albino rats by intraperitoneal administration of STZ (50 mg/kg.b.w).for 30 days. total cholesterol (TC), triglycerides (TG), very low density lipoprotein (VLDL), low density lipoprotein (LDL) and high density lipoprotein (HDL) cholesterol were estimated. There was a significant decrease in the activities of liver and renal functional markers in diabetic treated rats compared to untreated diabetic rats.

- Singh et al., (2013) investigated the modulation of liver function, antioxidant responses, insulin resistance and glucose transport by Oroxylum indicum stem bark in STZ induced diabetic rats. to administration of 65 mg/kg streptozotocin (STZ) for 28 days. In vivo effects of oroxylum indicum (OI) extract (oral 250 mg/kg b.wt.) on STZ induced type II diabetic rats normalized the antioxidant status (p ≤ 0.01) Lowering of total cholesterol and HDL levels (p ≤ 0.05) and restoration of glycated Hb (p ≤ 0.01) were also found in OI treated diabetic rats.

⬥   **Vikas Kumar et al., (2013)** Investigated anti-diabetic, anti-oxidant and anti-hyperlipidemia activities of *Melastoma malabathricum (MM)* Linn. leaves in streptozotocin induced diabetic rats. Diabetes was induced in rat by single intra-peritoneal injection of streptozotocin (55 mg/kg) for 28 days. Streptozotocin induced diabetes groups rat treated with different doses of MM leaves extract and glibenclamide significantly increased the body weight. Suggests a potential therapeutic treatment to antidiabetic conditions.

⬥   Ramesh R Petchis et al., (2013) evaluated antidiabetic and antihyperlipidemic effects of an ethanolic extract of the whole plant of *Tridax procumbens (Linn.)* in streptozotocin-induced diabetic rats Wistar rats by streptozotocin (50 mg/kg, i.p.) and nicotinamide (120 mg/kg, i.p) injection. The dry mass of the extract was used for preliminary phytochemical and pharmacological analysis. Diabetic rats were treated with glibenclamide (0.25 mg/kg, p.o.) or *T. procumbens* extract (250 and 500 mg/k, p.o.) for 21 consecutive days. The blood samples were collected at regular intervals to access hypoglycemic effect of an ethanolic extract of the whole plant *of T. procumbens*. At the end of the experiment, serum lipid profile and liver enzymes levels were analyzed for all the experimental animals and compared with diabetic control. The ethanolic extract of the whole plant of *T. procumbens* at 250 and 500 mg/kg has significant antidiabetic and antihyperlipidemic activities. The diabetic control animals exhibited a significant decrease in body weight compared with control animals. *T. procumbens* inhibited streptozotocin-induced weight loss and significantly alter the lipid.The preliminary phytochemical analysis of an ethanolic extract of the whole plant of *T. Procumbens* indicated the presence of alkaloids, tannins, flavonoids, saponins, and phenolic compounds. diabetic control animals showed significant increases of blood glucose levels (P<0.001). ethanolic extract of the whole plant of *T. procumbens* and glibenclamide-treated rats, but the diabetic control showed elevated SGPT, SGOT levels at the end of the experiment (P < 0.001).

⬥   Shahla Sohrabipour et al.,(2013) evaluated the effect of the administration of *Solanum nigrum* fruit on blood glucose, lipid profiles, and sensitivity of the vascular mesenteric bed to phenylephrine in streptozotocin-induced diabetic rats. to investigate the effect of the administration of oral doses of saqueous extract from *Solanum nigrum* fruit on plasma glucose, lipid profiles, and the sensitivity of the vascular mesenteric bed to Phenylephrine in diabetic and non-diabetic rats.caused Ca/Mg ratio, plasma glucose, high-density lipoprotein (HDL), low-density lipoprotein (LDL), very low-density lipoprotein (VLDL), total cholesterol, and triglyceride concentrations to return to normal levels, and was shown to decrease alteration in vascular reactivity to vasoconstrictor agents. Solanum nigrum administration in the ND-SNE group (1.29±0.07) caused the plasma magnesium level to decrease significantly (P<0.001) in comparison to the NDC group.

⬥ David et al.,(2012) Investigated the antihperglycemic activity of methanol extract of *Acorus calamus* (AC) rhizome. Male albino rats were rendered diabetic by Streptozotocin (STZ) (40 mg/kg i.p.) was determined orally to diabetic rats for 21 days. Results show that AC methanol extract possess potent antihyperglycemic activity in normal and STZ induced diabetic rats.

⬥ Santiagu et al., (2012) Investigated the antidiabetic and antioxidant effects of *Toddalia asiatica* leaves in Streptozotocin (STZ) 40mg/kg b.wt. induced diabetic rats. antidiabetic and antioxidant activities were studied for the ethyl acetate extract. Results of the experiments showed that Toddalia asiatica leaves ethyl acetate extract exerted significant antidiabetic and antioxidant effe cts in STZ-induced diabetic rats.

⬥ J et al.,(2012) evaluation of antidiabetic activity and chemical characterization of aqueous /ethanol prop roots extracts of Pandanus fascicularis Lam in streptozotocin-induced diabetic rats Diabetes was induced in rats by intra peritoneal (i.p) injection of STZ at a dose of 60mg/kg body weight. Preliminary phytochemical screening revealed the presence of carbohydrates, proteins, aminoacids, saponins, tannins, phenolic compounds, alkaloids and flavonoids,and the reduced blood glucose level was significant (P < 0.001) in the dose of 250 mg/kg of ethanol and aqueous extracts of P. fascicularis, when compared with control.

⬥ Gandhi et al., (2012) Studied antidiabetic effect of methanolic extract of (100, 200 and 400mg/ kg) of *Merremia emarginata* in streptozotocin induced diabetic rats for dose dependent effects of 28 days.

⬥ Naskar et al.,(2011) Investigated the effect of antidiabetic activity and effect on lipid profile as well as cardioprotective effect of hydro-methanol extract of *Cocos nucifera* (HECN) on streptozotocin (STZ)-induceddiabetic rat.

⬥ Salahuddin et al., (2010) Investigated antidiabetic activity of aqueous fruit extract of Cucumis *trigonus* Roxb (Cucurbitaceae) on streptozotocin-induced-diabetic40mg/kgfor 28 days. Cucumis trigonus showed beneficial effects in reducing the elevated blood glucose level and lipid profile of STZ-induced-diabetic rats.

Murugesan Gnanadesigan et al .,(2011) evaluated the hepatoprotective and antioxidant properties of marine halophyte *Luminetzera racemosa* bark extract in CCL_4 induced hepatotoxicity. Wistar albino rats were divided into 6 groups: Group 1 served as control; Group 2 served as hepatotoxin (CCL_4 treated) group; Group 3 served as positive control (Silymarin) treated groups; Group 4, 5 and 6 served as (100, 200 and 300 mg/kg bw p.o.) *L. racemosa* bark extract treated the hepatoprotective and antioxidant activities of the bark extract might be to the presence of unique chemical classes such as flavonoids, alkaloids and polyphenols. level of serum glutamate oxyloacetic transaminase (SGOT), serum glutamic pyruvic transaminase (SGPT), alkaline phosphatise (ALP), bilurubin, cholesterol, sugar and lactate dehydrogenase (LDH) were significantly ($P<0.05$) increased in hepatotoxin treated rats.

Jittawan Kubola et al., (2011) investigated the phytochemicals, vitamin C and sugar content of Thai wild fruits The objective of the present study was to generate information about the potential health-enhancing properties of selected Thai wild fruits. Nineteen varieties of wild fruits, collected from the natural forest in north-eastern Thailand, were analysed for phytochemicals, anti-oxidant activity, vitamin C and sugar content. The results showed that *Diospyros decandra* Lour. exhibited the highest content of total phenolic compounds (215 mg GAE/g) and total flavonoid content (187 mg RE/g). *Terminalia chebula* Retz had higher anti-oxidant activities than other fruits, as measured by 1,1-diphenyl-2-picrylhydrazyl radical scavenging (99% inhibition) and ferric reducing/anti-oxidant power assays (63 mmol $FeSO_4$/g). The sum of sugars (sucrose, glucose, fructose and galactose) ranged from 33 to 430 mg/g fresh weight, being dominated by glucose (ranging from 7.5 to 244 mg/g) and fructose (ranging from 5.3 to 193 mg/g).). The highest content of vitamin C was found in *Phyllanthus emblica* Linn. (2.2 mg/g). Thai wild fruits, which were investigated in this study, have been shown to be a novel rich source of phytochemicals.

Wintola et al., (2011) evaluated the Phytochemical constituents and antioxidant activities of the whole leaf extract of *Aloe ferox* Mill 1,1- diphenyl-2-picrylhydrazyl (DPPH), 2,2'-azino-bis(3-ethylbenzthiazoline-6-sulfonic acid) (ABTS) diammonium salt, hydrogen peroxide (H_2O_2), nitric oxide (NO), lipid peroxidation and ferric reducing power. Total phenols, flavonoids, flavonols, proanthocyanidins, tannins, alkaloids and saponins were also determined using the standard methods.

⬥ Jaouhari et al., (1999) investigated the hypoglycemic activity of *Zygophyllum gaetulum* extracts in alloxan-induced hyperglycemic rats. tested orally (1 g:kg body weight) for hypoglycemic activity in alloxan-induced diabetic rats. The infusion was partitioned between water and butanol to yield a butanol soluble fraction (B), and an aqueous fraction (W) which on reduction in volume gave apiecipitate (WP) and supernatant (WS). Fractions (B) and (WP) caused significant reduction in blood glucose concentration, while the ingestion of (WS) produced no significant reduction in blood glucose level (5).

⬥ Bhuvaneswari et al.,(2012) evaluated nephroprotective effects of ethanolic extract of *Sesamum indicum* seeds (Linn.) in streptozotocin induced diabetic male albino rats,65mg/kg for8 weeks. STZ-induced diabetic rats showed a significant decrease in the levels of serum total protein, albumin and globulin and significant increase in the levels of blood urea, serum creatinine and uric acid when compared to normal rats. These levels were reverted after the treatment regimen.

⬥ Asad et al., (2011) investigated the *Acacia Nilotica* Leave Extract and Glyburide: Comparison of Fasting Blood Glucose, Serum Insulin, b-Thromboglubulin Levels and Platelet Aggregation in Streptozotocin Induced Diabetic Rats administering 50 mg/kg body weight (b.w) streptozotocin and was confirmed by measuring fasting blood glucose level >200 mg/dL on 4th post-induction day. The rats were equally divided into 4 groups, A (normal control), B (diabetic control), C (diabetic rats treated with AN extract) and group D (diabetic rats treated with glyburide). The rats of group C and D were given 300 mg/kg b.w AN extract and 900 µgm/kg b.w glyburide respectively for 3 weeks. Blood glucose was measured by glucometer, platelet aggregation by Dia-Med method and insulin and b-thromboglobulin by ELISA technique. Leaves extract result into hypoglycaemic and anti-platelet aggregation activity in diabetic rats as that of glyburide. significant increase (p<0.05) in fasting blood glucose, b-thromboglobulin and platelet aggregation and a significant decrease (p<0.05) in insulin levels was observed in streptozotocin induced diabetic rats than the normal controls.

⬥ Petchi et al., (2013) evaluated antidiabetic and antihyperlipidemic effects of an ethanolic extract of the whole plant of *Tridax procumbens (Linn.)* in streptozotocin-induced diabetic rats. Diabetes was induced in male Wistar rats by streptozotocin (50 mg/jk, i.p.) and nicotinamide (120 mg/kg, i.p) injection. The dry mass of the extract was used for preliminary phytochemical and pharmacol ogical analysis. Diabetic rats were treated with glibenclamide (0.25 mg/kg, p.o.) or *T. procumbens* extract (250 and 500 mg/k, p.o.) for 21 consecutive days. The blood samples were collected at regular intervals to access hypoglycemic effect of an ethanolic extract of the whole plant of *T. procumbens*. At the end of the experiment, serum lipid profile and liver enzymes levels were analyzed for all the experimental animals and compared with diabetic control. The diabetic control animals exhibited a significant decrease in body weight compared with control animals. *T. procumbens* inhibited streptozotocin-induced weight loss and significantly alter the lipid levels.

Venkateshwarlu et al.,(2013) evaluation of anti diabetic activity of carica papaya seeds on streptozotocin- induced Type-II diabetic rats. At a dose of 100 mg/kg, 200mg/kg the extract was given to Male Sprague- Dawley rats for 14 days to evaluate the anti hyperglycemic and anti hyperlipidaemic activity in streptozotocin nicotinamide induced diabetic rats. Glibenclamide was used as a standard drug determined. Dosage of 100mg/kg and 200mg/kg of the extract significantly ($P<0.001$, $P< 0.01$) decreased blood glucose levels and the decrease was found to be dose dependent. SGOT, SGPT levels were decreased ($P<0.01$, $P<0.05$). Lipid profile was also decreased significantly ($P<0.01$, $P<0.05$).

❖ Chattopadhyay et al.,(2005) investigated the effects of *Azadirachta indica* leaf extract on serum lipid profile changes in normal and streptozotocin -induced diabetic rats have been studied with a view to elucidate its possible effect on cardiovascular disease induced by hyperglycemia. It was observed that *A. indica* leaf extract significantly reduced the total cholesterol, LDL- and VLDL-cholesterol, triglycerides and total lipids of serum in streptozotocin induced diabetic rats but HDL-cholesterol levels remained unchanged when compared with streptozotocin- induced diabetic control animals.

2.6 GLIBENCLAMIDE Increases insulin binding and sensitivity at receptor sites, stimulating insulin release from beta cells in pancreas and reducing blood glucose level. Also decreases production of basal glucose in liver, enhances sensitivity of peripheral tissue to insulin, inhibits platelet aggregation, and causes mild diuresis.

Contraindications

• Hypersensitivity to drug,• Type 1 (insulin-dependent) diabetes,Severe renal, hepatic, thyroid or other endocrine disease,• Pregnancy or breast feeding,

Precautions *Use cautiously in: **mild to moderate hepatic, renal, or cardiovascular disease; impaired thyroid, pituitary, or adrenal function infection, stress,***

Adverse reactions *CNS:* dizziness, drowsiness, headache, weakness,CV: increased CV mortality risk ,EENT: visual accommodation changes, blurred vision.,I: nausea, vomiting, diarrhea, constipation, cramps, heartburn, epigastric distress, anorexia,Hematologic: aplastic anemia, leukopenia, thrombocytopenia, agranulocytosis, pancytopenia ,Hepatic: cholestatic jaundice, hepatitis,Metabolic: hyponatremia, hypoglycemia,Skin: rash, pruritus, urticaria, eczema, erythema, photosensitivity, angioedema.

2.6.1 Herbal drugs in diabetes :

Indian herbal drugs and plants used in the treatment of diabetes,especially in india.In india it is proving to be a major health problem.Though there are various approaches to reduce the ill effects of diabetes and its secondary complications, herbal formulations are preffered due to lesser side effects and low cost.Many common herbs and spieces are claimed to have blood sugar lowering properties that make them useful for people with or high risk of type 2 diabetes. The clinical studies of Aloe vera have been carried out to recent herbal therapies and shown an improved blood glucose control in diabetes.

OBJECTIVE OF THE STUDY:

Collection and authentication of plant and the plant parts.

Extraction of plant material with 50% ethanol by cold percolation method.

To induce diabetes in experimental animals with Streptozocin.

To carry out the extensive pharmacological studies of *Spondias pinnata* extract in order to find out the efficacy against antidiabetic activity.

To investigate the biochemical parameters.

RESEARCH ENVISAGED:

Scientific literature indicating that *Spondias pinnata* is useful in various ailments such as antihelmentic, hypoglycaemic, hepatoprotective, antidiarrheal.The various parts of *Spondias pinnata* reported for various pharmacological activities while the antidiabetic activity has not been investigated in detail, which provides enough scope for further investigation. Antihypoglycaemic activity of *S. pinnata* against alloxane induced diabetes have been reported (Mondal et al.,2009).however, no investigative reports exist pertaining to its antidiabetic activity on STZ induced diabetes in experimental rats, hence the present study is designed to demonstrate the antidiabetic effect of *Spondias pinnata* against streptozotocin induced diabetes in experimental rats.

Chemicals and Drugs

All the chemicals which were used are of analytical grade, and they are listed below in a Table. 4.1.

Table 4.1. Chemicals and Drugs

A) Drugs & chemical

Normal Saline	Albert David Ltd, Ghaziabad
Streptozocin	Sigma Chemicals, USA (BCBF6608V), China
Glibenclamide	Loba Chemie pvt ltd.
Diethyl ether	S.D. Fine Chemicals, Mumbai, India
Formaldehyde	S.D. Fine Chemicals, Mumbai, India
Methanol	Fisher scientific Ltd, Mumbai, India
Ethanol	Changshen Yanguan Chemical, china

B) Enzymatic Kits

ALT (GPT) Test Kit	Span diagnostics ltd, Surat (76LS200-60)
AST Test ki	Span diagnostics ltd, Surat
Urea Test Kit	Span diagnostic ltd, Surat (71LS200-60)
Total Protein Test Kit	Span diagnostic ltd, Surat (83LS100-600)
Creatinine Test Kit	Span diagnostic ltd, Surat (71LS200-60)
Alkaline Phosphate Test Kit	Span diagnostic ltd, Surat (75DP200-50)

C) Equipments

U.V.Spectrophotometer (Double Beam)	Pharmaspec UV-1700, Shimadzu
Micropipette (10-100 µl & 100-1000 µl)	Superfit
Centrifuge	Almicro Micromeasures & Instruments
Digital Balance	ShimadzuAUX 220 Unibloc(PAT1987)
Refrigerator	Intello Cool LG.

Collection and authentication of plant materials

The fruits of *Spondias pinnata* (Anacandeacae) were collected from local market of Lucknow, in the month of January 2014. The plant material was authenticated by Mr. Muhmmad Arif (Assistant Professor) and Dr. Arshan Hussain (Associate Professor) Department of Pharmacognosy and Phytochemistry, Faculty of Pharmacy, Integral University, Lucknow- 226 022, A voucher specimen of *Spondias pinnata* (Anacandeacae) . (IU/PHAR/HRB/14/12) was deposited in the institute for further reference.

47

Preparation of extract

The freshly collected friuts of *Spondias pinnata* (Anacandeacae) was washed with distilled water to remove dirt and soil and shade dried. Dried plant material was removed peel small pieces and reduced to coarse powder by mechanical grinder and further extraction was carried out with 50 % hydroalcoholic by cold percolation method to avoid damage due to heat. The extract was filtered and concentrated under reduced pressure below $40 \pm 1°C$ using roteva vaccum rotary evaporator (Model no- UDOIAB-2391 Medica instrument) to dryness to get a constant weight. The % yield was found to be 18% w/w. The extract was stored in -20 °C freezer and used for Pharmacological investigation.

Phytochemical investigation (Kokate et al.,1994)

Various extracts of sample were subjected to Qualitative chemical tests for determinig the presence and type of phytoconstituents.

Test for alkaloids : Test for alkaloids was done by following method

- ☐ Mayer's test: Alkaloids give cream colour precipitate with Mayer's reagent [potassium mercuric iodide solution].
- ☐ Dragandroff's test: Alkaloids give reddish brown precipitate with Dragandroff's reagent [potassium bismuth iodide solution].
- ☐ Wagner's test: Alkaloids give a reddish brown precipitate with Wagner's reagent [solution of iodine in potassium iodide].
- ☐ Hager's test: Alkaloids give yellow colour precipitate with Hager's reagent [saturated solution of picric acid].
- ☐ Tannic acid test: Alkaloids give buff colour precipitate with 10% tannic acid solution.

Test for glycosides

- ☐ General test for the presence of Glycosides:

Part A:

Extracted 200 mg of the drug by warming in a test tube with 5ml of dilute (10 %) sulfuric acid on a water bath at 100°C for 2 min, centrifuge or filter, pipette off supernatant or filtrate. Neutralize the acid extract with 5 % solution of Sodium hydroxide (noting the volume of NaOH added). Added 0.1 ml of Fehling's solution A and then B until alkaline (test with pH paper) and heat on a water bath for 2min. Noted the quantity of red precipitate formed and compare with that formed in Part - B.

Part B:

Extracted 200 mg of the drug using 5ml of water instead of sulfuric acid. After boiling add volume of water equal to the volume of NaOH used in the above test. Add 0.1ml of Fehling's solution A and B until alkaline (test with pH paper) and heat on water bath for 2 min. Noted the quantity of red precipitate formed.

Compared the quantity of precipitate formed in Part-B with that of formed in Part-A. If the precipitate in Part-A was greater than in Part-B then Glycoside may be present. Since Part-B represents the amount of free reducing sugar already present in the crude drug. Whereas Part-A represents free reducing sugar plus those related on acid hydrolysis of any sides in the crude drug.

The extract is tested for free sugar:

Chemical tests for specific glycosides:

Test for saponin glycosides:

a) Froth Test: Placed 1 ml solution of drug in water in a semi-micro tube shake well and note the stable froth.

Test for anthraquinone glycosides

☐ Borntrager's test:

Boiled test material with 1ml of dil. sulphuric acid in a test tube for 5 min (anthracene glycosides are hydrolyzed to aglycone and sugars by boiling with acids) centrifuge or filter while hot (if centrifuged hot, the plant material can be removed while anthracene aglycones are still sufficiently soluble in hot water, they are however insoluble in cold water), pipette out the supernatant or filterate, cool and shake with an equal volume of dichloromethane (the aglycones will dissolve preferably in dichloromethane) separate the lower dichloromethane layer and shake with half its volume with dilute ammonia. A rose pink to red color is produced in the ammonical layer (aglycones based on anthroquinones give red color in the presence of alkali).

b) **Modified Borntrager's test:**

Boiled 200 mg of the test material with 2 ml of dilute sulphuric acid, 2 ml of 5 % aqueous ferric chloride solution for 5 min and continued the test as above. As some plant contain anthracene aglycone in a reduced form, if ferric chloride was used during the extraction, oxidation to anthroquinones took place, which showed response to the Borntrager's test.

Test for cardiac glycosides:

☐ Keller-killiani test [test for Deoxy sugars]:

Extracted the drug with chloroform and evaporated it to dryness. Added 0.4 ml of glacial acetic acid containing a trace amount of ferric chloride. Transfered to a small test tube; added carefully 0.5 ml of concentrated sulphuric acid by the side of the test tube, blue color appears in the acetic acid layer if cardiac glycoside was present.

Test for tannins& phenolic compounds:

Tannins and phenolic compounds were confirmed present if the following test were positive.

    a. Gelatin test:

Extract with 1 % gelatin solution containing 10% sodium chloride gives white precipitate.

    b. Ferric chloride test:

Test solution gives blue green color with ferric chloride.

    c. Vanillin Hydrochloride test :

Test solution when treated with few drops of vanillin hydrochloride reagent gives purplish red color.

    d. Tannins get precipitated in the solution when treated with heavy metals.

    e. Tannins yield bulky precipitate with phenazone specially in the presence of sodium and phosphate.

    f. Alkaline reagent test :

Test solution with sodium hydroxide solution gives yellow to red precipitate within short time.

Test for flavonoids:

Flavanoids were assumed to be present, if following tests were positive.

    a. Shinoda test (magnesium hydrochloride reduction test):

To the test solution add few fragments of magnesium ribbon and add conc. hydrochloric acid drop wise, pink scarlet, crimson red or occasionally green to blue color appears after few minutes.

    b. Zinc hydrochloride reduction test:

To the test solution add a mixture of zinc dust and conc. hydrochloric acid. It gives red color after few minutes.

    c. Alkaline reagent test:

To the test solution add few drops of sodium hydroxide solution; formation of an intense yellow color, which turns to colorless on addition of few drops of dil. acid, indicates presence of flavonoids.

Test for sterols & triterpenoids:

Steroids and triterpenoids were assumed to be present, if following tests were positive.

a. Libermann-Bruchard test:

Extract treated with few drops of acetic anhydride, boil and cool, conc. Sulfuric acid is added from the sides of the test tube, shows a brown ring at the junction of two layers and the upper layer turns green which shows the presence of steroids and formation of deep red color indicates the presence of triterpenoids.

b. Salkowski test:

Treat extract in chloroform with few drops of conc. sulfuric acid, shake well and allow to stand for some time, red color appears at the lower layer indicates the presence of steroids and formation of yellow colored lower layer indicates the presence of triterpenoids

Test for carbohydrates:

Carbohydrate was assumed to be present, if following tests were positive.

a. Molisch's test: Treated the test solution with few drops of alcoholic alpha naphthol Add 0.2 ml of conc. sulfuric acid slowly through the sides of the test tube, a purple to violet colour ring appears at the junction.

b. Benedict's test:

Treated the test solution with few drops of Benedict's reagent (alkaline solution containing cupric citrate complex) and upon boiling on water bath, reddish brown precipitate forms if reducing sugars are present.

c. Barfoed's test:

It is a general test for monosaccharide. Heat the test tube containing 1 ml of reagent and 1ml of solution of compound in a beaker of boiling water; if red cuprous oxide is formed within 2 min, monosaccharide is present. Disaccharide on prolonged heating (about 10 min) may also cause reduction, owing to partial hydrolysis to monosaccharides.

d. Tollen's test:

To 100 mg of compound add 2ml of Tollen's reagent and heat gently, a silver mirror is obtained inside the wall of the test tube, indicates the presence of aldose sugar.

e.Bromine water test:

It gets decolorized by aldose but not by ketoses because bromine water oxidizes selectively the aldehyde group to carboxylic group, giving raise to general class of compounds called aldonic acid.

f.Fehling's test:

Equal volume of Fehling's A (copper sulfate in distilled water) and Fehling's B (potassium tartarate and sodium hydroxide in distilled water) reagents are mixed and few drops of sample is added and boiled, a brick red precipitate of cuprous oxide forms, if reducing sugars are present.

Animals:

Adult male Wistar rats weighing 160 - 200 g were procured from National Laboratory Animal Center, Central Drug Research Institute (CDRI), Lucknow. They were kept in departmental animal house, Integral University. The animals were housed separately in polypropylene cages for acclimitization at a temperature of (23 ± 2 °C) and 50–60% relative humidity, with a 12 hr light/dark cycle one week before and during the commencement of the experiment. Animal were kept on standard pellet diet (Dayal animal feed, Unnao, India) and drinking water *ad libitum* throughout the housing period. Administration of the extract and toxicant was done by oral route in the morning session throughout the study period. All experimental procedures involving animals were conducted in accordance with the guidelines of Committee for the Purpose of Control and Supervision on Experiments on Animals (CPCSEA). The study protocols were approved by the Institutional Animal Ethics Committee (IAEC) of Integral University, Faculty of Pharmacy, Lucknow, India (Reg. no. 1213/GO/ac/08/CPCSEA).

Experimental Schedule for Antidiabetic Activity

The animals were randomly be assigned into 5 groups of 5 animals each and receive the following treatments: Group I: Normal control + distilled water, Group II: Diabetic, Group III: Diabetic + *Spondias pinnata* extract peel (SPE) (50 mg/kg), Group IV: diabetic + drug (100mg/kg), Group V: Diabetic + drug (150mg/kg) and Group VI: Diabetic + Glibenclamide (10mg/kg). The freshly prepared solutions was orally administered daily for 15 days. Diabetes will be induced by single intra-peritoneal injection of 55 mg/kg of streptozotocin (STZ), freshly dissolved in cold citrate buffer, pH 4.5. After 3 days of STZ injection, animals with fasting blood glucose above 250 mg/dL will be considered as diabetic and included in the study.

Groups	No. of rats	Treatment	Dose
I	5	Control + distilled water	10 ml/kg
Ii	5	STZ	55 mg/kg
Iii	5	STZ + SPE	100 mg/kg
Iv	5	STZ + SPE	200 mg/kg
V	5	STZ + Glibenclamide	10 mg/kg

After the last dose of SPE peel (i.e. 24 hours), blood samples of each animal was obtained as per CPCSEA guideline for estimation of various biochemical parameters and the animals will be sacrificed.

Parameters for investigation

Initial and final body weight: During the experiment 0, 7 and 14th day body weight were recorded.

Estimation of Blood glucose level. (Arunachalam et al.,2013)

Collection of blood samples

Blood samples were collected from the retro -orbital plexus of rats under anesthesia at 1, 7, 14, days intervals. Blood was collected in heparinized tubes (eppendorf) and used for the estimation of bloo d glucose level by Accu Check.

Assessment of biochemical analysis:

Plasma alanine transaminase (ALT), Alkaline Phosphate (ALP), Total protein, urea, and Creatinine was determined by using standard kits from Span diagonistic ltd, Surat, India. All estimation was carried out using UV spectrophotometer (Shimadzu, india) as per standard kit methods. The estimation procedure is obtained in detail from leaflets provided by the commercially available kits are as follows.

Alanine aminotransferase (ALT) [GPT] test kit
Modified UV (IFCC), kinetic assay, Span Diagnostic Ltd. (Liquid Gold), Surat.

Alanine aminotransferase (ALT) also know as glutamate pyruvate transaminase (GPT) is a transaminase. The highest levels are found in the liver and in kidneys, and in smaller amount in heart and skeletal muscle.

Assay Principle

Alanine aminotransferase (ALT) catalyses the transamination of L-Alanine and α-ketoglutarate to form Pyruvate and L-Glutamate. In subsequent reaction, Lactate Dehydrogenase (LD) reduces Pyruvate to Lactate with simultaneous oxidation of Nicotinamide Adenine Dinucleotide [reduced] (NADH) to Nicotinamide Adenine Dinucleotide (NAD). The rate of oxidation of NADH is measured kinetically by monitoring the decrease in absorbance at 340 nm. LD rapidly and completely reduces the endogenous sample Pyruvate during the initial incubation period, so that it does not interfere with the assay.

Working Reagent Preparation

Add reagent 2 to reagent 1 in 1:4 ratio i.e., 1 mL of Reagent 2 + 4 mL of Reagent 1.

Assay Parameters

Mode	Kinetic
Reaction direction	Decreasing
Wavelength	340 nm
Flow- cell temperature	37° C
Optical path length	1 cm
Blanking	Purified water
Sample volume	100 µL
Reagent volume	1000 µL
Delay	60 seconds
Interval	30 seconds
Number of reading (s)	4
Permissible Reagent Blank absorbance	>1.0 AU
Kinetic factor	1768
Maximum ΔA/minute	0.26
Linearity	450 IU/L
Units	IU/L

Procedure

Pipette into tube marked	**Test**
Serum/Plasma	100 µL
Working ALT Reagent	1000 µL

Mix well and aspirate immediately for measurement.

Programme the analyser as per assay parameters.

1. Blank the analyser with Purified Water.

2. Read absorbance after 60 seconds. Repeat readings after every 30 seconds i.e., upto 120 seconds at 340 nm wavelength.

3. Determine the mean absorbance change per minute (ΔA/minute).

Calculation

ALT Activity (IU/L) = ΔA/minute x kinetic factor

Where

ΔA/minute = change in absorbance per minute

Kinetic factor (K) = 1768

Kinetic factor is calculated by using following formula

$$K = 1/M \times TV/SV \times 1/P \times 10^6$$

M = Molar extinction coefficient of p-Nitrophenol and is equal to 1.8×10^3 lit/mol/cm at 405 nm

TV = Sample volume + Working Reagent volume

SV = Sample volume

P = Optical path length

10^6 = Constant

Clinical Significance

Serum AST and ALT levels are elevated in viral and other forms of liver diseases associated with Hepatic necrosis. ALT is more liver specific enzyme.

Increased activity: Serum activity of ALT is increased in Liver diseases, in Trauma or in Skeletal disease after Renal infract and in various Haemolytic conditions. In Viral Hepatitis associated with necrosis the elevation would be 20 to 50 fold, peak values reaching between 7th and 12th day returns to normal levels in 3 to 5 weeks in uneventful recovery. In Alcoholic Hepatitis there is moderate elevation. In Viral Hepatitis ALT levels are increased even before appearance of Jaundice. ALT levels may be raised without elevated Serum Bilirubin in condition known as Anicteric Hepatitis. The levels remain slightly elevated even after disappearance of clinical Jaundice. Moderate increase may be seen in Cirrhosis, Extrahepatic Cholestatis and Carcinoma of Liver.

Alkaline phosphatase test kit

pNPP-AMP (IFCC), Kinetic Assay, Span Diagnostic Ltd. (Liquid Gold), Surat.

Assay Principle

At pH 10.3, Alkaline Phosphatase (ALP) catalyses the hydrolysis of colourless p-Nitrophenyl Phosphate (pNPP) to yellow coloured p-Nitrophenol and Phosphate. Change in absorbance due to yellow colour formation is measured kinetically at 405 nm and is proportional to ALP activity in the Sample.

p-Nitrophenyl Phosphate + H$_2$O $\xrightarrow{\text{ALP}}$ p-Nitrophenol + Phosphate

Assay Parameters

Mode	Kinetic
Wavelength	Increasing
Flow- cell temperature	37°C
Optical path length	1 cm
Blanking	Purified water
Sample volume	20 μL
Reagent volume	1000 μL
Delay	30 seconds
Interval	30 seconds
Number of reading(s)	4
Permissible reagent Blank absorbance	<0.1 AU
Kinetic factor	2712
Maximum ΔA/minute	0.36
Linearity	Upto 1000 IU/L
Units	IU/L

Procedure

Pipette into tube marked	**Test**
Serum/ Plasma	20 μL
Working ALP Reagent	1000 μL

Mix well and aspirate immediately for measurement

Programme the analyser as per assay parameters.

1. Blank the analyser with Purified Water

2. Read absorbance after 30 seconds. Repeat reading after every 30 secinds i.e., upto 120 seconds at 405 nm wavelength.

3. Determine the mean absorbance change per minute (ΔA/minute).

Calculations

ALP activity (IU/L) = ΔA/minute x Kinetic factor

Where

ΔA/minute = Change in absorbance per minute

Kinetic factor (K) = 2712

Kinetic factor is calculated using following formula

$$K= 1/M \times TV/SV \times 1/P \times 10^6$$

M = Molar extinction coefficient of p-Nitrophenol and is equal to 1.8×10^3 lit/mol/cm at 405 nm

TV = Sample volume + Working Reagent volume

SV = Sample volume

P = Optical path length

10^6 = Constant

Clinical Significance

Serum ALP measurement is of particular interest in the Hepatobiliary disease and is bone diseases. The main site of synthesis of this enzyme is hepatocytes adjacent to Biliary canaliculi and active osteoblast. However, it is known that response of a liver to any form of Biliary tree obstructuion is to synthesise more ALP.

Increased activity: Serum ALP is increased in diseases of bone including Metastasis, Rickets, Paget's disease and in healing fractures, Intrahepatic or Extrahepatic obstruction in Liver. Elevated levels are seen in growing Children due to new bone formation (Osteoblastic activity). Increase in ALP activity may often be the first indication of Hepatotoxic action of therapeutic drugs. Marked elevation in the absence of Jaundice but in the presence of primary source may be indicative of Metastasis.

Decreased activity: Low levels of ALP are found in a rare Congenital Defect, Hypophosphatasemia and in Pernicious Anemia.

Total protein test kit

Modified Biuret, End Point Assay, Span Diagnostic Ltd. (Liquid Gold), Surat.

Assay Principle

The peptide bonds of proteins react with Cupric ions in alkaline solution to form a coloured chelate, the absorbance of which is measured at 578 nm. The Biuret Reagent contains Sodium-Potassium Tartrate, which helps in maintaining solubility of this complex at alkaline pH. The absorbance of final colour is proportional to the concentration of Total Protein in the Sample.

$$\text{Protein} + Cu^{++} \xrightarrow{\text{Alkaline pH}} \text{Cu-Protein Complex}$$

Assay Parameters

Mode	End point
Wavelength	578 nm (550-580 nm)
Flow- cell temperature	37°C
Optical path length	1 cm
Blanking	Reagent Blank
Sample volume	10 μL
Reagent volume	1000 μL
Incubation time	5 minutes

Concentration of standard	6.5 g/dL
Stability of final colour	2 hours

Permissible reagent Blank absorbance	<0.2 AU
Linearity	Upto 20 g/dL
Units	g/dL

Procedure

Pipette into tube marked	Blank	Standard	Test
Serum / Plasma	-	-	10 μL
Reagent 2	-	10 μL	-
Reagent 1	1000 μL	1000 μL	1000 μL

Mix well. Incubate at 37°C for 5 minutes.

Programme the analyser as per assay parameters.

1. Blank the analyser with reagent Blank

2. Measure absorbance of the Standard followed by the Test.

Calculation

Total Protein concentration (g/dL) = Absorbance of Test/ Absorbance of Standard X 6.5

Globulins = Total Protein – Albumin

Conversion factor

Total Protein concentration in g/L = Total Protein concentration in g/dL X 10

Clinical Significance

Total Protein estimate is useful for monitoring gross changes in protein levels caused by various disease states.

Increased concentration: Dehydration, Monoclonal diseases (Myeloma, Macroglobulinemia, Cryoglobulinemia) and some chronic Polyclonal diseases, (Liver Cirrhosis, Sarcoidosis, Systemic Lupus Erythematosis).

Decreased concentration: Over hydration, Protein loss through Kidneys (Nephrotic syndrome), from Skin (Severe Burns), Starvation, Protein Malnutrition, severe Non Viral Liver cell damage.

Urea test kit

Span Diagnostic Ltd. (Liquid Gold), Surat.

64

Assay Principle

Enzymatic determination according to the following reactions.

$$\text{Urea} + 2H2O \xrightarrow{\text{Urease}} 2NH4 + CO3$$

$$NH4 + \alpha\text{-Ketoglutarate} + NADH \xrightarrow{\text{GLDH}} L\text{-Glu} + NAD + H2O$$

Assay Parameters

Mode	2 point
Wavelength	340 nm
Flow- cell temperature	37°C
Sample volume µl	10 µL
Reagent volume µl	1000 µL
Delay	30 seconds
Interval	90 seconds
Concentration of standard	50 mg/dl
Linearity	300 mg/dl
Ref. low	13
Ref.high	43
Units	Mg/dl

One reagent procedure

	Blank	Standard	Sample
Reagent R	1000 µL	1000 µL	1000 µL
Standard	-	10 µL	-
Sample	-	-	10 µL

Mix after 30 seconds at 37 ºC,measure A1.After 90 secondsfurther measure.

	Blank	Standard	Sample
Reagent R 1	400 µL	1000 µL	1000 µL
Reagent R 2	100 µL	10 0µL	100 µL

Mix and wait 25 seconds.

	Blank	Standard	Sample

Standard		5 µL	
Sample			5 µL

Mix after 30 seconds at 37 ºC, measure A1. After 90 seconds further measure A2($\Delta A = A2 - A1$).

Procedure

Mixed well and aspirate immediately for measurement

Programmed the analyser as per assay parameters.

1. Blank the analyser with Purified Water

2. measured A1.After 90 seconds further measure A2(ΔA=A2-A1).

Calculations

ΔA sample/ΔA standard × n

Where

n = standard concentration

Take the dilution factor into account for the calculation of urea concentration in urine.

Creatinine test kit

Modified jaffe's reaction, initial rate Assay, Span Diagnostic Ltd. (Liquid Gold), Surat.

Assay

Principle

Creatinine react with picric acid in an alkaline medium to form an orange colored complex. The rate of formation of this complex is measured by reading the change in absorbance at 505 nm in a selected interval of time and is proportional to the concentration of creatinine. The reaction time and the concentration of picric acid and sodium hydroxide have been optimized to avoid interference from ketoacids.

Creatinine + Picric acid ——— Alkaline medium   orange coloured complex

Assay Parameters

Mode	Initial Rate
Wavelength	505 nm(490-530nm)
Flow- cell temperature	37°C
Optical path length	1 cm
Blanking	Purified water
Sample volume	100 µL
Reagent volume	1000 µL
Delay	30 seconds

Interval	120 seconds
Number of reading(s)	1
Permissible reagent Blank absorbance	<0.35 AU
Concentration of standard	2mg/dl
Linearity	Upto 20 mg/dl

Reaction direction	Increasing
Units	Mg/dl

Pipette into tube marked	Standard	Test
Serum / Plasma/Urine	-	100 µL
Reagent 3	100 µL	-
Working Creatinine Reagent	1000 µL	1000 µL

Procedure

Mixed well and aspirate immediately for measurement

Programmed the analyser as per assay parameters.

1. Blank the analyser with Purified Water

2. Measured initial absorbance of the standard i.e.AS1 after 30 seconds and final absorbance (AS2) after an interval of another 120 seconds.

3. After standard reading are noted, take the reading of Test i.e. AT1 and AT2

Calculations

Serum/Plasma creatinine (mg/dl)= AT2-AT1/AS2-AS1×2

Urine Creatinine (mg/day)= AT2-AT1/AS2-AS1×2×dilution factor ×24 hrs urine volume in dL.

AT1 = Initial O.D.of Test

AT2 = Final O.D.of Test

AS1 = Initial O.D.of standard

AS2 = Final O.D. of Standard

Clinical Significance

Creatinine is an end product formed in muscles from creatine Phosphate, the high energy storage compound.creatinine production primarily a function of muscle .mass and the amount produced is fairly constant.creatinine is removed from plasma by glomerular filtration and is then excreted in urine. Therefore, creatinine clearance is a measure of glomerular filtaration rate (GFR) and its measurement is useful in assessing renal function.serum cretinine is more specific and sensitive indicator of renal function than serum urea. The urine / plasma creatinine ratio is greater than 40 in pre-renal uremia and less than 20 in renal uremia.

Increased concentration

The concentration of serum creatinine rises when there is impaired formation or excreation of urine ,irrespective of whether the causes are pre-renal ,renal or post renal in origin.

Decreased concentration

Low serum creatinine has no clinical significance.

5.1 Effect on body weight

Body weight gain in vehicle control group after 14 days was recorded from 180.5 to 191.45. Diabetes prevents the weight gain on 7th day and 14th day from 178.6 to 171.16 and 171.6 to 162.42 in group II respectively. SPE (100 and 200 mg/kg) treated groups showed non significant decrease in body weight gain on 7th day and 14th day respectively (Table 5.2). Standard drug treated group showed significant increase ($P < 0.05$ to $P < 0.01$) in body weight gain.

Table 5.2

Showing the chemical tests of various extracts of *Spondias* Pinnata.

S.NO	EXTRACT	METHANOL	CHLOROFORM	PETROLEUM ETHER	ETHYL ACETATE
1.	Alkaloid	+ve	-ve	-ve	+ve
2.	Amino acid	ve	-ve	-ve	ve
3.	Steroid/Tri-terpenoids	-ve	-ve	-ve	-ve
4.	Tannins	+ve	-ve	-ve	+ve
5.	Flavanoid	+ve	-ve	-ve	+ve
6.	glycosides	+ve	-ve	-ve	+ve
7.	Reducing sugar	+ve	-ve	-ve	-ve
8.	Saponin	+ve	-ve	-ve	+ve

Effect on serum blood glucose

Fasting blood glucose levels were determined on zero day, 7th day and 14th day which is described in Table 5.3. Blood glucose levels in the diabetic group II increased significantly from the initial day to the termination of experimental period ($P < 0.001$) in comparison to vehicle control group. SPE in dose of 100 and 200 mg/kg has nonsignificant effect on blood glucose level when compare to STZ group II rats. However, Glibenclamide treated rats showed significant reduction ($P<0.001$) in blood glucose level throughout the study period in comparison with diabetic group II rats.

Effect on biochemical parameters

The results of biochemical parameters were described in table 5.4. STZ induced diabetes has significantly increased the serum level of AST ($P < 0.01$), ALT ($P < 0.001$), ALP ($P < 0.01$), urea ($P < 0.001$) and creatinine ($P < 0.001$) level in animals compared to vehicle control group I. Effect of SPE at 200 mg/kg dose on serum AST ($P < 0.05$), ALT ($P < 0.05$), ALP ($P < 0.05$) and urea ($P < 0.05$) were decreased significantly while the dose of SPE at 100 and 200 mg/kg shows significantly decrease in creatinine level ($P < 0.05$ to $P < 0.01$) when compared to STZ group II rats (Table 5.4) indicating that the kidney protective activity of the selected plant.

Table 5.2 Effect of *Spondias pinnata* extract on body weight against streptozotocin (STZ) induced diabetic in experimental groups of rats.

Groups	Treatment	Body weight (g)		
		0 day	**7th day**	**14th day**
I	Control	180.5 ± 19.84	184.56 ± 15.26	191.45 ± 14.23
II	STZ 55 mg/kg, i.p.	178.6 ± 16.21	171.16 ± 18.59	$162.42 \pm 11.41^{\#}$
III	SPE 100 mg/kg + STZ	164.5 ± 14.73	159.81 ± 18.54	151.08 ± 10.78^{ns}
IV	SPE 200 mg/kg + STZ	175.8 ± 17.45	170.33 ± 17.85	161.22 ± 12.45 ns
V	Glibenclamide 10 mg/kg	177.9 ± 20.77	$183.57 \pm 13.28^{*}$	$190.27 \pm 13.52^{**}$

Values are expressed as mean $\pm$ SEM of 5 rats in each group.

P values: [#]<0.001 compared with respective normal control group I

P values: [*]<0.05, [**]<0.01 and ns (Non significant) compared with group II (STZ).

Table 5.3 Effect of *Spondias pinnata* extract on blood glucose level against streptozotocin (STZ) induced diabetic in experimental groups of rats.

Groups	Treatment	Blood glucose level (mg/dL)		
		0 day	**7th day**	**14th day**
I	Control	91.4 ± 18.5	86.5 ± 17.4	88.5 ± 17.6
II	STZ 55 mg/kg, i.p.	$437.4 \pm 21.1^{\#}$	$453.1 \pm 33.2^{\#}$	$471.1 \pm 32.7^{\#}$
III	SPE 100 mg/kg + STZ	426.4 ± 31.3^{ns}	438.7 ± 34.2^{ns}	439.8 ± 28.4^{ns}
IV	SPE 200 mg/kg + STZ	411.8 ± 32.6^{ns}	425.8 ± 27.4^{ns}	432.3 ± 27.8^{ns}
V	Glibenclamide 10 mg/kg	$90.41 \pm 12.36^{*}$	$81.9 \pm 16.3^{*}$	$73.5 \pm 13.3^{*}$

Values are expressed as mean ± SEM of 5 rats in each group.

P values: $^{\#}<0.001$ compared with respective normal control group I

P values: *<0.001 and ns (Non significant) compared with group II (STZ).

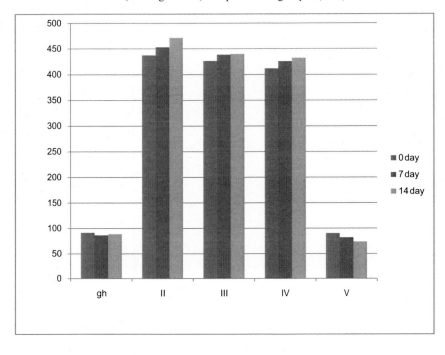

Table 5.4 Effect of *Spondias pinnata* extract on biochemical parameters against streptozotocin (STZ) induced diabetic in experimental groups of rats.

Groups	AST (U/L)	ALT (U/L)	ALP (U/L)	Urea (mg/dL)	Creatinine (mg/dL)
I	90.13 ± 8.6	37.53 ± 5.38	81.22 ± 7.86	24.36 ± 1.3	0.87 ± 0.12
II	$128.36 \pm .8.2^{\#}$	$92.53 \pm 8.81^{\#\#}$	$138.29 \pm 10.24^{\#}$	$63.42 \pm 3.2^{\#\#}$	$2.48 \pm 0.13^{\#\#}$
III	117.16 ± 9.45^{ns}	81.78 ± 7.59^{ns}	108.25 ± 8.51^{ns}	51.12 ± 2.8^{ns}	$1.96 \pm 0.14^{*}$
IV	$105.81 \pm 9.45^{*}$	$65.28 \pm 6.18^{*}$	$98.43 \pm 8.27^{*}$	$39.31 \pm 2.1^{*}$	$1.12 \pm 0.11^{**}$
V	$89.33 \pm 8.52^{**}$	$43.45 \pm 7.23^{**}$	$80.24 \pm 7.52^{**}$	$28.61 \pm 2.4^{***}$	$0.96 \pm 0.09^{***}$

Values are expressed as mean $\pm$ SEM of 5 rats in each group.

P values: $^{\#}<0.01$, $^{\#\#}<0.001$ compared with respective control group I

P values: $^{*}<0.05$, $^{**}<0.01$, $^{***}<0.001$ and ns (Non significant) compared with group II (STZ).

Diabetes mellitus is one of the leading causes of death, illness and economic loss all over the world. Whereas insulin-dependent (type I, IDDM) diabetes is characterized by juvenile onset and by absolute insulin deficiency, non-insulin-dependent (type II, NIDDM) diabetes is characterized by mature onset, by varying basal insulin levels and a frequent association with obesity. It is likely that further heterogeneity exists within these two basic types. Similarly, animal models of diabetes differ significantly from each other and none of them can be taken, without reservations, to reproduce the essentials of human diabetes (Bell and Hye, 1983).

STZ is a valuable agent for the production of diabetes because it allows the consistent production of diabetic states with mild, moderate, or severe hyperglycemia, where animals with mild or moderate diabetes have provided an opportunity to study the influence of oral hypoglycemic agents, and STZ-induced diabetic rats have been widely used as a model for diabetes mellitus in experimental animal (Murphy and Anderson 1974).

In this study, hypoglycemic effect of ethanolic extract of *Spondias pinnata* was evaluated by assessing body weight change, blood sugar level and related biochemical parameters. Obesity is mostly associated with diabetes mellitus, indicating weight control as an important aspect of diabetes management. Our results showed that all the animals treated with SPE have lost weight during the study period. The weight loss was highest in the diabetic control group II while Glibenclamide treated group showed weight gain.

The diabetic control group II animals showed fasting blood glucose level above 250 mg/dl, which has remained higher throughout the study period of 14 days. Glibenclamide (10 mg/kg) was used as a standard drug, showed decrease in blood glucose level from the initial to termination of the experiments. The SPE in all treated doses showed nonsignificant change in blood glucose level throughout the study period indicated that selected plant is ineffective in antidiabetic activity.

Glibenclamide has effective reduced the elevated liver enzymes and creatinine level in diabetic animals. In the present study it was found that significant reduction in serum glutamate oxaloacetate transaminase (SGOT) level along with serum glutamate pyruvate transaminase (SGPT) and alkaline phosphatase (ALP) level by the alcoholic extract of *Spondias pinnata* (200 mg/kg) signifying its hepatoprotective effect. (Hazra et al.), *Spondias pinnata* has been traditionally claimed for its hepatoprotective activity and during this investigation we found the same effect this indicates protective effect of SPE on liver either by reducing oxidative damage or by normalizing liver lipid metabolizing and turnover mechanism.

In this study, urea and creatinine was significantly increased in diabetic group II and Glibenclamide effectively control all these disturbed parameters. SPE treated group showed significant change in serum urea and creatinine level. Kidney maintains optimum chemical composition of body fluid by acidification of urine and removal of metabolic wastes such as urea, uric acid, creatinine, and ions. During renal diseases, the concentration of these metabolites increases in blood (Virdi et al., 2003).

- In this study, the diabetic animals showed significantly higher level of serum creatinine, which has been reduced to normal by SPE at 100 and 200 mg/kg dose treatment. This effect may be due to the diuretic action of *Spondias pinnata* ethanolic extract as reported by (Arunachalam et al.,2013). Normalization of creatinine level by SPE indicates that it has protective effect on the kidney and further studies are required to explore the effect of SPE on kidney. The SPE in all treated doses showed absence of antidiabetic effect indicating no effect on β-cells of the pancreas or not related to increased utilization of glucose by cells. On many cases beneficial flavonoids are less effective due to poor solubility, decreased bioavailability, first pass metabolism and intestinal degradation (Mohan et al., 2014).

Mondal et al., 2009 evaluated for hypoglycemic activity of *Spondias pinnata* bark on adult Wistar albino rats at dose levels of 300 mg/kg p.o. each using normoglycaemic, glucose loaded and alloxan induced for 14 days. Glibenclamide (2.5 mg/kg) was used as reference standard for activity comparison. Among the tested extracts, the methanol extract was found to produce promising results that is comparable to that of the reference standard glibenclamide. The results of the study justify the use of the barks of the plant for treating diabetes as suggested in the folklore remedies.

During this study the effect of *Spondias pinnata* peel extract on Streptozotocin induced diabetes in rats showed absence of antidiabetic activity while Mondal et al., 2009 reported antihyperglycemic effect of *Spondias pinnata* bark extract against Alloxan induced diabetes in rats.

7.1 CONCLUSION

The result from this study does not support the usage of this plant as a beneficial practice in folk medicine in the treatment of diabetes. The effect of *Spondias pinnata* peel extract was not significant on hyperglycemia induced by Streptozotocin, but it has significant effect on normalization of liver enzyme and serum creatinine level indicating possible presence of liver and kidney protective property.

American Diabetes Association. Standards of medical care in diabetes ., 2012. *Diabetes Care*. 35 Suppl 1:S11-63.

Alemzadeh R,Wyatt DT.,2007. Diabetes mellitus. In Kliegman RM, ed. Nelson Textbook of Pediatrics. 18th edition. Saunders; pp. 590.

Anita K., 2012.Medicinal plants against snake envenomation. International journal, 3 :(3).

Arunachalam K, Parimelazhagan.,2013. , evaluated the effect of methanolic extract of the bark of Ficus amplissim on streptozotocin-induced diabetic rats. Journal of Ethanopharmacology, pp. 302-310.

Asad M, Munir A, Afzal N.,2011.Investigated the Acacia Nilotica Leave Extract and Glyburide: Comparison of Fasting Blood Glucose, Serum Insulin, b-Thromboglubulin Levels and Platelet Aggregation in Streptozotocin Induced Diabetic Rats. journal of Pakistan medical Association, .pp.88-94.

Badoni A, Bisht C., 2009. Importance and Problems in Natural Regeneration of Spondias pinnata. (5):12-13.

Barik R., 2008. Antidiabetic activity of aqueous root extract of Ichnocarpus frutescens in streptozotocin-nicotinamide induced type-II diabetes in rats. Indian Journal Pharmacology, 40(1): 19–22.

Bell RH, Hye RJ (1983) Animal models of diabetes mellitus: physiology and pathology. J Surg Res 35:433–460.

Bhuvaneswari P , Krishnakumar S., 2012. Evaluated Nephroprotective effects of ethanolic extract of Sesamum indicum seeds (Linn.) in streptozotocin induced diabetic male albino rats. 6 :330-335.

Chakrabarti, S., Biswas, T.K., 2005. Antidiabetic activity of Caesalpinia bonducella F. in chronic type 2 diabetic model in Long-Evans rats and evaluation of insulin secretagogue property of its fractions on isolated islets. Journal of Ethnopharmacology, 97: 117–122.

Chattopadhyay R,Bandyopadhyay M., 2005. Effects of Azadirachta indica leaf extract on serum lipid profile changes in normal and streptozotocin -induced diabetic rats. African s journal of Biomedical research, 8 :101-104.

Chhetri, D.R., Parajuli, P., 2005. Antidiabetic plants used by Sikkim and Darjeeling Himalayan tribes. Indian Journal of Ethnopharmacology. 99: 202-199.

David H, Rangachari.B., 2012. Antidiabetic activity of methanol extract of Acorus calamus in STZ induced diabetic rats. Asian Pacific Journal of Tropical Biomedicine, pp.941-946.

Eliza J, Daisy P., 2010.Antioxidant activity of costunolide and eremanthin isolated from Costus Biological Interactions. Journal of Ethnopharmacology, 188:467–472

.Ghate N.B., 2013. In vitro anticancer activity of Spondias pinnata bark on human lung and breast carcinoma. Springer Science, pp.1-2.

Gnanadesigan M, kumar S, Inbaneson J., 2011.Evaluated the hepatoprotective and antioxidant properties of marine halophyte Luminetzera racemosa bark extract in CCL4 induced hepatotoxicity. Asian Pacific Journal Tropical Medicine. pp.462-465.

Goodman and Gilman's.,2008.manual of pharmacology and therapeutics,Vol.11 edition,pp.1037-1058.

Hazra B, Biswas S., 2013. Antioxidant and free radical scavenging activity of Spondias pinnata.

,BMC Complement Altern.med,12: 123-133.

.Kamboj A.,2008. Diabetes mellitus or impaired glucose tolerance.Diabetology,pp.201-203.

Hazra B, Biswas S., 2013. Antioxidant and free radical scavenging activity of Spondias pinnata.

,BMC Complement Altern.med,12: 123-133

.Kamboj A.,2008. Diabetes mellitus or impaired glucose tolerance.Diabetology,pp.201-203.

Jaouhari J.T , Lazrek H.B.,1999. the hypoglycemic activity of Zygophyllum gaetulum extracts in alloxan-induced hyperglycemic rats. Journal of Ethnopharmacology ,pp. 17–20.

Jittawan K,Sirithon S, Naret M., 2011. Investigated the phytochemicals, vitamin C and sugar content of Thai wild fruits ,Journal of ethanopharmacology, Pages 972–981.

K. Raju, R Balaraman.,2008. Antidiabetic mechanisms of saponins of Momordica cymbalaria Pharmacognosy Magzine, 4: pp. 115-113.

Kesari AN, Kesari S.,2007. Studies on the glycemic and lipidemic effect of Murraya koenigii in experimental animals. Journal Ethnopharmacology, 112: 305-311.

Katzung B,Masters S,Trevor A.,2009.Basic and clinical pharmacology, Vol.11 edition,pp.727-749.s

Kirtikar K.R, Basu B.D., 1935. Indian Medicinal Plants. Lalit Mohan Basu Publications, pp.

1139–1141

.Kokate, C.K., 1994. Practical Pharmacognosy. Vallabh Prakashan, New Delhi, 105–107.

Kumar R., 2013. Antihyperglycemic effect of Eugenia jambolana seed kernel on streptozotocin-induced diabetes in rats. Food Chemical Toxicology, 43, 1433 -1439.

Kumar V, Ahmed D, Gupta P, Anwar F, and Mujeeb M.,2013. Investigated anti-diabetic, anti-oxidant and anti-hyperlipidemia activities of Melastoma malabathricum (MM) Linn. leaves
82

in streptozotocin induced diabetic rats. BMC complimentary and alternative medicine,pp.1472-6882.

Latha, M, Pari L., 2004. Effect of an aqueous extract of Scoparia dulcis on blood glucose, plasma insulin and some polyol pathway enzymes in experimental rat diabetes. Brazilian Journal of Medical and Biological Research, 37, 577–586.

Mohan SN. Role of various flavonoids: Hypotheses on novel approach to treat diabetes. Journal of Medical Hypotheses Ideas 2014;8:1-6.

Mondal S, Dash G K., (2009). Hypoglycemic activity of the bark of Spondias pinnata. 5: 42-45.

Murphy ED, Anderson JW.,1974. Tissue glycolytic and gluconeogenic enzyme activities in mildly and moderately diabetic rats: Influence of tolbutamide administration. Endocrinology 94:27-34.

Nabi S, Kasett R , Sirasanagandla S, Tilak, Malaka T, Kuma V, Rao C., *BMC complementary and alternative medicine*, 13: 37-40.

Naik, V.R, Agshikar N.V., 1981. Cucumis trigonus Roxb. II. Diuretic activity. Journal of Ethnopharmacology, 3: 15–19.

Naskar S, Pramanik G, Gupta M, Kumar S., 2012. Evaluation of antihyperglycemic activity of Cocos nucifera Linn. on streptozotocin induced type 2 diabetic rats. Journal of ethnopharmacology, (3):769-763.

Panda S, Patra N.,2012.Antidiarrheal activity.International journal medicine,2: 123-134.

Pari .L ,Rajarajeswari N., 2009. Efficacy of coumarin on hepatic key enzymes of glucose metabolism in chemical induced type 2 diabetic rats. Biological Interactions Journal of Ethnopharmacology, 181: 292–296.

Petchi R, Parasuraman S., 2013. Evaluated antidiabetic and antihyperlipidemic effects of an ethanolic extract of the whole plant of Tridax procumbens (Linn.) in streptozotocin-induced diabetic rats .4: 88-92.

Ramos R., 2012. Antioxidant and anti-inflammatory effects of a hypoglycemic fraction from Cucurbita ficifolia Bouché in streptozotocin-induced diabetes mice. 40:97-110.

Salahuddin M, Jalalpure S., 2010. Antidiabetic activity of aqueous fruit extract of Cucumis trigonus Roxb. In streptozotocin-induced diabetic rats. Journal of Ethnopharmacology, pp.565–567.

Shahla Sohrabipour , kharazmi F,Soltani,Kamalinejd M., 2013. evaluated the effect of the administration of Solanum nigrum fruit on blood glucose, lipid profiles, and sensitivity of the vascular mesenteric bed to phenylephrine in streptozotocin-induced diabetic rats.Medical science monitor basic research, 19:133-140.

Singh J, Kakkar P.,2013. modulation of liver function, antioxidant responses, insulin resistance and glucose transport by oroxylum indicum stem bark in stz induced diabetic rats . Food and Chemical Toxicology,volume 62:722-731.

Stephen S .,2012. Antidiabetic and antioxidant activities of Toddalia asiatica leaves in Streptozotocin induced diabetic rats. Journal of Ethnopharmacology, pp. 515–523.

Tandon, S, Rastogi R.P., 1976. Studies on the chemical constituents of Spondias pinnata, Planta Med, 290, 180.

Tripathi K,2013.Essentials of medical pharmacology,Vol.7 edition,pp.258-281.

Venkateshwarlu E, Dileep P, Kumar R, Sandhya P .,2013.evaluation of anti diabetic activity of carica papaya seeds on streptozotocin- induced Type-II diabetic rats. Journal of Advanced Scientific Research, pp203.

Virdi J, Sivakami S, Shahani S, Suthar AC, Banavalikar MM, Biyani MK. Antihyperglycemic effects of three extracts from Momordica charantia. J Ethnopharmacol 2003;88:107-711.

Wintola.O, Anthony Jide Afolayan ., 2011. Evaluated the Phytochemical constituents and antioxidant activities of the whole leaf extract of *Aloe ferox* Mill 1,1- diphenyl-2-picrylhydrazyl (DPPH), 2,2'-azino-bis(3-ethylbenzthiazoline-6-sulfonic acid) (ABTS) diammonium salt, hydrogen peroxide (H2O2), nitric oxide (NO), lipid peroxidation and ferric reducing power. Pharmacognosy magazine,Vol.7,pp.325-333.

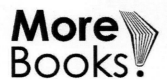
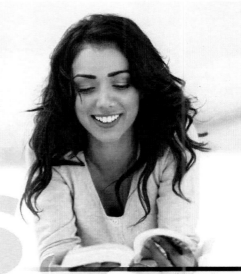
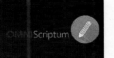